Sexuality and Fertility Issues
in Ill Health and Disability

of related interest

Third Party Assisted Conception Across Cultures
Social, Legal and Ethical Perspectives
Edited by Eric Blyth and Ruth Landau
ISBN 1 84310 084 3 (paperback)
ISBN 1 84310 085 1 (hardback)

Experiences of Donor Conception
Parents, Offspring and Donors through the Years
Caroline Lorbach
Foreword by Eric Blyth
ISBN 1 84310 122 X

Counsellors in Health Settings
Edited by Kim Etherington
Foreword by Tim Bond
ISBN 1 85302 938 6

An A-Z of Community Care Law
Michael Mandelstam
ISBN 1 85302 560 7

Sexuality
Your Sons and Daughters with Intellectual Disabilities
Karin Melberg Schwier and Dave Hingsburger
ISBN 1 85302 896 7

Sex, Sexuality and the Autism Spectrum
Wendy Lawson
Foreword by Glenys Jones
ISBN 1 84310 284 6

Sexuality and Women with Learning Disabilities
Michelle McCarthy
Foreword by Hilary Brown
ISBN 1 85302 730 8

The Chronic Illness Game
Isabelle C. Streng and A.M. Stradmeijer
Board game ISBN 1 84310 376 1

Understanding 12–14-Year-Olds
Margot Waddell
ISBN 1 84310 367 2

Parenting Girls
Janet Irwin, Susanna de Vries and Susan Stratigos Wilson
ISBN 1 85302 946 7

Special Brothers and Sisters
Stories and Tips for Siblings of Children with a Disability or Serious Illness
Edited by Annette Hames and Monica McCaffrey
Illustrated by Brendan McCaffrey
ISBN 1 84310 383 4

Sexuality and Fertility Issues in Ill Health and Disability

From Early Adolescence to Adulthood

Edited by
Rachel Balen and Marilyn Crawshaw

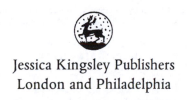

Jessica Kingsley Publishers
London and Philadelphia

Front cover artwork: *Arrow* by Dan Savage
'The arrow to the left-hand side of this piece depicts the arrow that was drawn on my leg for the operation. That such a rudimentary method was employed by the doctors prior to a major operation seemed to me to be rather basic. As I found out more information about my condition, I began to reflect on my own life. This self-reflection is symbolized by the use of a mirrored surface behind the figure's head. I pored through biology textbooks, medical websites and leaflets to try to find out as much as I possibly could. The diagrams in the piece, together with the morphing of the figure into a biological diagram, are representative of this time.

This piece is also concerned with a consequence of the chemotherapy that I was unprepared for. The quick onset of chemotherapy meant that I had to be rushed through sperm banking. The background is the consent form that I had to sign. Not only was I experiencing incredible embarrassment at the time but I also had to consider decisions that I would be making in years to come – about starting a family. Suddenly the realization that I might be affected long term made me think of the wider implications of chemotherapy.'

First published in 2006
by Jessica Kingsley Publishers
116 Pentonville Road
London N1 9JB, UK
and
400 Market Street, Suite 400
Philadelphia, PA 19106, USA

www.jkp.com

Copyright © Jessica Kingsley Publishers 2006

The right of the contributors to be identified as authors of this work has been asserted by them in accordance with the Copyright, Designs and Patents Act 1988.

Library of Congress Cataloging in Publication Data
Sexuality and fertility issues in ill health and disability : from early adolescence to adulthood / edited by Rachel Balen and Marilyn Crawshaw.
p. cm.
Includes bibliographical references and index.
ISBN-13: 978-1-84310-339-4 (pbk. : alk. paper)
ISBN-10: 1-84310-339-7 (pbk. : alk. paper) 1. Youth with disabilities--Sexual behavior. 2. Sex (Psychology) 3. Sex instruction for people with disabilities. 4. Sex instruction for the sick. 5. Sex counseling. 6. Fertility. I. Balen, Rachel, 1954- II. Crawshaw, Marilyn, 1949-
HQ30.5.S235 2006
306.7087--dc22

2006000753

British Library Cataloguing in Publication Data
A CIP catalogue record for this book is available from the British Library

ISBN 13: 978 1 84310 339 4
ISBN 10: 1 84310 339 7

Printed and bound in Great Britain by
Athenaeum Press, Gateshead, Tyne and Wear

For Josh and Geoffrey

Acknowledgement

We would like to thank Sue Hanson from the Centre for Applied Childhood Studies, University of Huddersfield, UK, for her assistance in the preparation of this manuscript.

Contents

Introduction

The teenage years, arguably more than any others, are marked out by a strong need to identify closely with same-age peers. As we move out from the world of childhood, where our reference group is primarily our family, the desire to look to those around us for the norms of how to behave, what to wear and what to do is increasingly dominant. Teenagers test the boundaries and experiment with the beckoning world of adulthood. Difference is taboo – except where it involves dreams of fame and fortune!

Within this context, growing up with the differences attached to physical impairment or a health condition can bring particular challenges. While caregivers – whether professionals, family or friends – may continue to try to meet physical needs, their ability to meet emotional and psycho-social needs will inevitably become more limited. They are simply no substitute for being 'one of the crowd'. When differences attach to some of the most intimate parts of our emerging identities – sexual and fertile identities – then the potential dangers to well-being are manifold.

This book is underpinned by the principle that young people living with impairments or health conditions are first and foremost young people. Their dreams and aspirations, contradictions and confusions, ups and downs need to be firmly located within the normality of their life stage. However, denying the potential impact of their condition on their experiences does them a disservice every bit as discriminatory as seeing the impairment rather than the person. Jenny Morris (2002) reminds us: 'Young disabled people have the same aspirations as their non-disabled peers but require specific action to tackle the disabling barriers that they experience.' If we fail to engage with the need to dismantle the barriers that get in the way of addressing sexuality and fertility for young people living with impairments or health conditions, then we fail to offer them the chance to feel good about themselves and to achieve socially and psychologically healthy adult identities. When adults fail to raise these intimate matters, the message is reinforced that they are 'better hidden' or, as Melissa Cull writes in Chapter 12, 'shrouded in shame and secrecy.'

We come to this work through our professional backgrounds in social work but also through our personal experiences – Rachel as the mother of a childhood cancer survivor now in his teens and Marilyn whose brother died from cancer as a young adult. Many of the authors similarly draw on their personal as well as professional experience. The range of disciplines represented here is also deliberate. The need to better understand and respond to sexuality and fertility issues is not restricted to any one professional discipline, context or country. Hence we have chapters from different parts of the first world and from social workers, nurses, gynaecologists, paediatricians, paediatric oncologists, scientists, psychologists, educators and researchers – the list could have been added to endlessly. Many conditions affect sexuality and fertility – too many to cover here – but readers will find much that is transferable across conditions as well as aspects that are unique. Finally, we have included the voices of those directly affected from a personal perspective.

The structure of the book

While there is an increasing literature that acknowledges sexuality in adults with physical impairments or health conditions, there is a marked lack of writing about childhood or adolescent sexuality and fertility issues. Contrast this to the burgeoning industry that surrounds teenage sexual health but which uses a narrow definition of sexual risk-taking and limited underpinning understanding of teenage sexuality and results in a concentration on pregnancy avoidance and reduction in sexually transmitted diseases. A glance at this and at school sex education curricula might lead one to conclude that there is no such thing as a teenager facing fertility difficulties! Little work has been done to enable us better to comprehend what those in middle childhood and teenage years understand about fertility and aspire to most as they become adults.

This book seeks to consider the ways in which teenagers and young adults manage their emerging sexuality when there is the possibility or probability that their fertility is impaired.

Part One: Children and young people's understanding of sexuality, fertility and parenting

This first section sets the context for the book. In Chapter 1, Sarah Andrews takes us through a whirlwind tour of the way that sexuality and sexual health is written about and understood. She raises challenging issues regarding the idea of children as sexual beings and how adults' reactions can be key in determining an individual's responses to his or her own sexuality and sexual health. Chapters 2 and 3 draw on a fascinating research study conducted by Balen, Fraser and Fielding, which explored children and young people's life ambitions, their ideas about becoming parents themselves and their understanding of the concept of (in)fertility. Their findings and the words of the young people themselves illuminate the world from which the teenager or young adult coping with sexuality and fertility issues has emerged.

Part Two: Medical, scientific, legal and ethical aspects of compromised fertility in adolescence and early adulthood

If formal and informal caregivers are to be alert to sexuality and fertility issues, then they need to be appropriately informed about current medical and scientific knowledge. Not surprisingly, many will be daunted by trying to understand the terminology, let alone weighing up the scientific merits of claims that hit the headlines on a regular basis.

This section draws on leading UK experts to pull together some of the key facts and messages about sexual and fertility difficulties that may attach to different conditions (Chapter 4 by Balen and Glaser) and different fertility preservation treatments that are available for females (Chapter 5 by Picton) and males (Chapter 6 by Pacey). The section concludes with a dip into the legal and ethical complexities that surround fertility preservation and reproductive medicine (Chapter 7 by Green and Crawshaw).

Part Three: Personal experiences of living with health conditions and disability and the impact on sexuality and fertility

The third section of the book aims to help the reader focus on the ways in which sexuality and fertility issues are experienced at a personal level by those on the pathway to adulthood.

Atkin, Rodney and Cheater (Chapter 8) remind us that some young people will already be coping with institutionalized and socially discriminatory attitudes and policies that, sadly, are still targeted at those from Black and minority ethnic communities. The need for services and policies to be on the alert for this is clear. Cull's chapter on intersex conditions (Chapter 12) and that of Cincotta, Childs and Eichenfield on HIV/AIDS (Chapter

13) reinforce the need to address the experience of discrimination that comes with being a 'member' of a stigmatized group, whether resulting from ethnicity, disability, a hidden and taboo health condition or any other source.

Several authors in this section have moved into professional careers in which they draw upon their personal experiences. Cull (Chapter 12) writes as a researcher and founder of a national support group, Zebrack (Chapter 14) uses his own young adult cancer experience to inform his research work with survivors while Self (Chapter 15), now a psychiatrist, writes poignantly of her journey to motherhood as a teenage cancer survivor.

Some of the conditions described are experienced from teenage years onwards while others are a lifelong experience. Teenage males newly diagnosed with cancer get catapulted into fertility decisions when faced with sperm banking and Crawshaw (Chapter 9) looks at their immediate and longer-term experiences. In contrast, Farrant and Sawyer (Chapter 11) explore the impact on young people who have lived with cystic fibrosis all their lives but increasingly face the implications of having impaired fertility. Cincotta, Childs and Eichenfield (Chapter 13) describe the impact of changes in attitudes as well as health interventions towards HIV/AIDS (in the Western world at least) over the lifetime of present-day teenagers and the care that they still have to take in knowing 'who to tell', while Loughlin (Chapter 10) works with young women with Turner Syndrome and reminds us of the need to create an environment for them in which to explore their sexuality and fertility but not necessarily through words.

Part Four: Voices

Our final section reflects the voices of young people, adults and parents who have been directly affected by the issues explored in this book. The contributors express their experiences through narrative, poetry and art and their words serve to remind readers of the importance of sexuality, (in)fertility and health in the lives of all of us.

Conclusion

We hope this book will encourage caregivers – professionals, family and friends – to be alert to this hitherto hidden part of growing up. But awareness is only the start. If we are to reduce any of the barriers that are there for these young people to emerge into adulthood feeling good about their sexual and fertility identities, this book suggests that they may need their caregivers to help them along the way. Not by trying to take the place of their peer group but by helping to enable them to take their place within that peer group with the confidence that comes with feeling that difference is not the same as deficiency.

Part One

Children and Young People's Understanding of Sexuality, Fertility and Parenting

1

Sexuality and Sexual Health Throughout the Childhood and Teenage Years

Sarah Andrews

Introduction

Any work with children and young people that concerns their fertility will have their sexuality and sexual health as a constant backdrop. Their understanding of what reduced fertility means and its effect on their lives as they grow towards adulthood will be influenced at least in part by how broader issues about sexuality and sexual health are dealt with by parents, carers and professionals. It is first and foremost essential to understand that sexuality forms part of our identity and experience from infancy onwards. An outline of how sexuality develops throughout the childhood and teenage years forms the first part of this chapter.

In the second part, sexual health and well-being will be considered. Some young people coping with health conditions and disability as they are growing up will also have to deal with adverse experiences such as sexual abuse, sexually transmitted infections, unwanted pregnancies and struggles with sexual identity.

The third part of this chapter will discuss the provision of age- and context-appropriate sexual health services and education. This includes the need to pay particular attention to the influence of disability or health conditions, whether or not the young person is accessing informal sources of information from their peers and/or formal sex education and whether or not they are sexually active. Issues of confidentiality are also addressed.

Finally, two important questions that need to be considered by parents and professionals will be discussed:

- How is this young person's sexuality affecting their behaviour, including what they are saying (or not) about their symptoms, feelings and relationships?

- How is the way this young person is being dealt with going to affect their future sexual health, sexual feelings and sexual relationships?

Development of sexuality and sexual identity

Sexuality is a dynamic concept and is about much more than sexual activity and sexual orientation alone. It includes what being male or female means to us and how we express our gender; how we feel about our bodies, about our appearance and about physical pleasure; whom we are attracted to and what we choose to do about it; and, if we have intimate relationships, how we behave with our partners. Our ability to reproduce comes from our sexual behaviour and our feelings about our sexuality and sexual identity can be deeply affected by our sense of our own fertility.

We are all born either male or female (with some exceptions covered in Chapter 12), with different chromosome patterns and body chemistry. From birth we are spoken to, handled and usually dressed differently as part of our socialization into our gender roles. As we grow up we learn how boys and girls are supposed to behave and our differing personalities and experiences leave us more or less comfortable with living up to these expectations. Some of these expectations and roles are based on the assumption that we will be parents in the future: for example, girls the world over may be given dolls with which to practise nurturing.

As we get older we learn the rules about when and where to cover up our private parts. These rules vary somewhat from culture to culture. The age at which these rules apply can differ even between siblings but at some point this is manifest by children becoming self-conscious about their bodies and desirous of privacy. The capacity for shame and embarrassment seems to be universal.

But are children sexual? Wilhelm Reich (1968) tells us that before the time of Sigmund Freud it was believed that 'Sexuality was something that, at the time of puberty, descended on the human out of a clear sky. "Sexuality awakens" so they said. Where it had been before, nobody seemed to know' (p.49).

The first widespread understanding of childhood sexuality began when Freud (1901) defined distinct developmental stages that children go through, with a sexual/pleasure focus being on a different part of their bodies in each stage. He labelled the first stage as oral, with pleasure gained through sensations in the mouth. The anal stage, during toilet training, comes next, then a phallic stage, from around ages three to five, as children first discover the pleasure of exploring their own genitals. Freud saw the middle childhood period (ages 5 to 12) as being a time of sexual latency, which is followed by the final mature genital stage, after puberty, when sexual feelings are directed towards other adults.

These stages have been used, contested and developed mainly within the field of adult psychotherapy (Bateman, Brown and Pedder 2000), but have been less used to aid understanding of children's sexual feelings, thoughts and behaviours. Freud's pronouncement that sexuality is 'latent' in the middle childhood years has led, in many cultures, to a lack of recognition of childhood sexuality (Ryan 2000). However, as Ryan points out, research across cultures has found evidence of considerable sexual activity and interest amongst pre-pubescent children. Her own American survey of adult child abuse professionals found that almost 20 per cent of respondents remembered experiencing sexual arousal by the age of six years (Ryan, Miyoshi and Krugman 1988).

It is clear that children of all ages, from infancy upwards, have the capacity to experience pleasure and reassurance from touching their genitals. Although there is wide variation between individuals, most girls and virtually all boys start to masturbate at some stage in their development. Some parents find this alarming and embarrassing and children may be told that touching themselves is wrong or 'naughty'. Scare stories told to children in the past to prohibit touching, such as 'It'll make you go blind' or 'You'll get hair growing on the palms of your hands', together with religious prohibitions, have had wide currency (Ryan 2000) and their legacy remains today in a general discomfort with the subject. Teaching children that private touching is for a private place (such as bathroom or bedroom) is a simple concept that helps children learn appropriate public behaviour without creating guilty feelings about sexual pleasure.

After falling for more than a century, the age at which puberty occurs has levelled off in many developed countries, both for boys and girls (see Chapter 4). Puberty in girls starts slowly with changes in body shape, but is usually marked by the onset of menstruation any time between the ages of 8 and 17, with the median age between 12 and 13 (Whincup *et al.* 2001). Boys start puberty slightly later than girls – at any time between 10 and 16 – but their body changes continue longer, until late teens or early twenties (Lee, Guo and Kulin 2001). While children with learning disabilities, physical disabilities and/or serious health conditions usually enter puberty at a similar age to their peers, they may have delayed emotional and social development that results in a need for extra help in understanding the changes they are experiencing (Hudson 2003).

The physical changes at puberty can bring changes in patterns of mood and emotions; for example, intense emotional attractions can be felt to adults of the same or opposite sex, such as pop stars, sporting stars and respected adults like teachers. This is part of the preparation for sexual relationships as sexual orientation becomes clearer. Sexual orientation is broader than whether we are attracted to males or females or both. It also covers other aspects of what we find attractive, including physical appearance and personality type, as well as any tendency for disordered attractions, such as towards children.

The average age of first sexual intercourse has gone down in many developed countries over recent years: in the UK the mean age is around 16 to 17 for both boys and girls (McCabe and Killackey 2004; Schubotz, Rolston and Simpson 2004). The age varies considerably between different groups in society, and those that start youngest are least likely to use contraception or safer sex the first time (Coleman and Roker 1998). There is much less information available about the age at which young people start to experiment with sexual activity other than intercourse, including with partners of the same sex, and it must be presumed that some of this will start earlier than intercourse.

Sexual health

Sexual health was defined by Mace, Bannerman and Burton (1974) as:

> a capacity to enjoy and control sexual and reproductive behaviour in accordance with social and personal ethics; freedom from fear, shame, guilt, false beliefs and other psychological factors inhibiting

sexual response and impairing relationships; freedom from organic disorders, diseases and deficiencies that interfere with sexual and reproductive functions. (p.10)

While other definitions have been explored since then, this one remains useful and comprehensive: it starts with the positive, then indicates factors that can damage sexual health unless preventive or remedial action is taken. Some examples of these factors are considered below.

Sexualized media images of children

Being surrounded by media images and a culture that glamorize physical perfection and sexualize the clothes and appearance of even very young children may make it difficult for children and young people to grow up feeling comfortable with their bodies. This may be especially so if they are different from the current ideal. For teenagers rehearsing their imminent adult identities, which will typically include a sexualized self-image, the pressures can be felt especially keenly.

Young people should be valued whatever their physical attributes. It is important to take opportunities to challenge stereotypes and to introduce a diversity of role models, so children learn that it is possible to be popular and attractive even if they look very different from catwalk models or pop stars.

Sexual abuse

Sexual abuse and exploitation of children and young people are now known to be widely prevalent. In 1978 Kempe defined child sex abuse as 'the involvement of dependent, developmentally immature children and adolescents in sexual activities that they do not fully comprehend, to which they are unable to give informed consent or that violate the social taboos of family roles' (p.382). However, as Haugaard (2000) points out, there continue to be ongoing debates about the definitions of the terms 'child', 'sexual' and 'abuse'.

What research there has been into the sexual development of pre-pubescent children has, in recent years, often been prompted by the need to identify abnormal behaviour as a sign of sexual abuse (Ryan 2000). Gail Hornor (2004) found that what is deemed to be 'normal' in child sexual behaviour is determined by the social, cultural and familial context of the times.

Marsha Heiman and colleagues (1998) urged professionals to be critically aware of how much their gender and their role may influence and inform their beliefs about what constitutes normal sexual behaviour in children, especially as it may be their judgement about what is considered to be age inappropriate sexual knowledge and behaviour that is a key criterion used to assess allegations of sexual abuse.

Susan Creighton (2004) reviewed international studies and found that, in the countries studied, despite variations in the definition of sexual abuse and in the recognition of the problem, between 8 and 42 per cent of girls and 3 to 25 per cent of boys had suffered from some kind of sexual abuse. Sex with children is illegal in most jurisdictions, although the age definition of 'child' may vary (Interpol 2005). Sex tourism, prostitution and child pornography affect millions of children around the world (Gallagher *et al.* 2003). Most sexual abuse, however, happens within families and it is often not reported. Children with disabilities are four to ten times more vulnerable to sexual abuse than other children and the perpetrators are often those involved in their care (Sobsey 1992).

Sexually transmitted infections (STIs)

STIs are on the increase, with many showing steep rises in recent years. Sexual intercourse without using a condom (outside of a life-long faithful partnership) brings the risk of an STI. Some STIs can be extremely serious, with complications leading to chronic disease, infertility and, in some cases, death. The global rise of HIV/AIDS is now widely recognized and the number of young people in the UK becoming infected with HIV through sexual intercourse is rising dramatically, amongst girls in particular (PHLS Aids Centre and the Scottish Centre for Infection and Environmental Health 2002). Other infections are, however, less commonly discussed. The prevalence of chlamydia, which can have severe effects on both male and female fertility, is now above one in ten in some parts of the world: the highest rates in the UK are amongst 16 to 19-year-old females and 20 to 24-year-old males (Health Protection Agency 2004a). Another very prevalent infection, human papillomavirus (HPV), can result in cervical cancer. Gonorrhoea and syphilis infections are increasing, sometimes in forms that resist treatment (Health Protection Agency 2004b, 2004c).

The only ways to protect against these infections are through monogamy, abstinence from penetrative sex or through the use of male or female condoms. STI clinics (sometimes called genitourinary medicine clinics or

GUM clinics) can advise about testing and treatment if an infection is suspected. Most young people will not be aware of the range or seriousness of these infections, or the need for specialist treatment. While some disabled young people have relatively high levels of contact with physicians, they rarely receive advice about how to avoid STIs (Surís *et al.* 1996). Young people with life-threatening conditions may be more likely to seek out risky behaviours, including risky sexual encounters, so could be at increased need of interventions to promote safer sex (Valencia and Cromer 2000).

Unwanted pregnancies

A consequence of sexual risk-taking for many young people will be an unplanned and possibly unwanted pregnancy. The UK has the highest rate of teenage pregnancy in Western Europe (UNICEF 2001). Many teenage pregnancies are wanted but the abortion figures give some indication of how many are not. In many countries, pregnancies in younger girls are more likely to end in abortion especially in more affluent socio-economic groups (Bradshaw 2002). Between 1999 and 2001 in the UK, 44 per cent of pregnancies in 15–19-year-olds resulted in abortions (Lee *et al.* 2004). Babies born to very young mothers are more at risk of health problems and may cause the mother's education to be interrupted, reducing her chances of future employment and leaving her and her child economically disadvantaged (Bradshaw 2002).

Young people whose condition or treatment may affect their current or future fertility may have ambivalent feelings about pregnancy and this, combined with the propensity for risky behaviour mentioned above, makes it essential that contraceptive options are raised carefully with teenagers who could be fertile. The range of suitable options should be covered, together with information about emergency (post-coital) contraception in case of accidents: no contraception is completely reliable.

Openness, sex education and sexual health services

Parents and teachers are often nervous about addressing the sensitive and potentially embarrassing subject of sex education. While some adults may fear that once young people know that sexual intercourse exists they will immediately rush off to try it, the evidence is to the contrary (Kirby 2002). Those countries that appear to offer the most effective sex education have the lowest teenage pregnancy rates and a higher average age for the start of sexual activity (Alan Guttmacher Institute 2001). Good sex education results in young people being more considered about sexual matters and more selective in their choice and number of sexual partners. DiCenso and colleagues (2002) confirmed that if the content of this education is wholly or predominantly biological, the outcomes are poorer. Curricula that are more broadly based and include 'sex and relationships education' or 'personal and social education' are more effective. The promotion of the idea of sexual abstinence until marriage may delay sexual activity but there has been little rigorous evaluation of formal abstinence programmes (Kirby 2001).

Sex education has some fundamental purposes that few would argue with: the protection brought by the acquisition of knowledge and skills; the need to prevent confusion, unhappiness and unnecessary shame or guilt; the aim of creating confidence, self-esteem and enjoyment of one's body; and the promotion of happy, successful and safe future relationships. However, active moral and religious debates mean that sex education content and methodology are influenced by wider factors.

There are perhaps three stages in children's lives in which they can be said to have distinct educational needs:

1. From the time that they start to walk and talk and through the middle childhood years, children are learning how to behave appropriately in public, including in relation to their bodies.

2. Children who are approaching puberty need to be prepared for the changes that this brings, both emotionally and socially – indeed some cultures have specific puberty-associated rites.

3. Those who have passed through puberty need to prepare for sexual relationships and for becoming adults.

For this reason, sex education is about much more than a one-off talk, rather it should be a continuing process which introduces new ideas at appropriate times in a child's life. Required topics for young children include:

- developing an understanding of the differences between male and female bodies

- understanding and applying the rules of their society about public and private behaviours relating to what body parts are kept covered, what touching is permitted and what behaviour is allowed in different places

- knowing the names for parts of the body, including private parts, so that they can report any problems such as pain, injury or unusual symptoms, which could indicate illness

- learning about 'good' and 'bad' touching and about 'good' and 'bad' secrets in order to reduce the potential for sexual abuse.

Before they reach puberty, children need to understand:

- what changes are about to happen to their bodies, including periods or wet dreams, and that these changes are a normal and healthy part of moving towards adulthood

- the changes that will happen to the bodies of children of the opposite sex and at least the basics of reproduction which needs to be conveyed alongside affirming messages that all bodies are different and that changes happen at different times for different individuals – sexual feelings and emotional changes can come to the fore during this time

- the 'rules' of their society about how, when and with whom to discuss these matters.

After puberty, young people need to know (although many would say that earlier teaching would be better):

- about personal relationships

- what sex is and how babies are made

- that it is wrong to have sex with a child, a close family member or with someone who does not want it

- that it is OK to say no to sexual advances, and how

- that some people are attracted to the same sex (some or all of the time)

- that contraception can prevent pregnancy

- about STIs and how to protect themselves

- that there are many different beliefs and views in society about sex, sexuality and sexual behaviour.

Much of this learning is picked up informally through interactions with parents, family, neighbours and friends (see Chapter 3). However, the accuracy and tone of what is absorbed in daily life is not always as clear or precise as it might be, so it is usual for parents and/or schools to teach at least some of the above in a more formal way. This of course needs to be tailored to the needs of individual children including those who may have had limited social interaction or those with learning disabilities. Formal sex education needs to combine provision of facts, understanding of feelings, learning about values and teaching of skills such as how to communicate about sexual matters.

The fear or experience of homophobia can affect the way that young people feel about themselves and express their sexuality. Homophobia means a fear or hatred of homosexuality that leads to expressions of discrimination or abuse. It can have its origins in personal or religious belief systems but can also be driven by insecurity and/or a desire to demonstrate one's own heterosexuality, especially in young men. Young people may experience discrimination and abuse if they are not, or appear not to be, heterosexual. Homophobia needs to be tackled just as much as do racism, sexism and other forms of discrimination. If it is not challenged then it will continue to adversely affect and limit all parts of society.

In addition to the provision of education, young people also need good quality, accessible services from health and social care professionals about sexual health, STIs, contraception and relationships. They have a right to confidential advice: anxiety about confidentiality can be a major deterrent to not seeking advice (Department of Health 2004a). One of the first reasons that young people contact health services independently is when they need emergency contraception or a pregnancy test. Young people may return repeatedly for emergency contraception or pregnancy tests and these visits can be used as opportunities for sexual health and/or relationships advice. This advice may not be acted on by the young person immediately but may form the basis of a positive advisory relationship for the future. Essential elements for sexual health services for young people include the core provision of reproductive health advice within accessible and young person-friendly settings where non-judgemental staff of both genders are available to offer advice and treatment to self-referred young people. Staff should be aware of issues of consent and competence, confidentiality and clinical care and there should be clearly defined routes of liaison with other child welfare services (Rogstad, Ahmed-Jushuf and Robinson 2002).

Kristin Luker's (1975) work on young people's contraceptive decisions identified that young people use a type of cost–benefit analysis in relation to their behaviour, with the short-term risks of having to admit to being sexually active and risking disapproval or loss of reputation sometimes far outweighing the more serious but distant risks of an STI or an unplanned pregnancy. Services thus have to work to ensure that their reputation for discretion and respect can overcome young people's anxiety and embarrassment. Professionals need to treat young people with respect and provide them with sufficient time and support to make informed choices about their existing and future sexual behaviour. The avoidance of a moralizing or paternalistic response is key (Department of Health 2004a).

Apart from the provision of education and services, parents, carers, educators and health and social care professionals need to provide the ingredients through which children and young people can develop a happy, healthy sexuality including:

- love, affection, respect and acceptance to help provide the young person with a strong sense of identity and self-esteem

- security and safety, which includes protection from exploitation and abuse as well as the chance to experiment and take risks in order to build resilience and future independence

- good relationship role-models within the family or wider social circles

- support for any developing relationships

- sources of advice, both within and outside the family environment, with the understanding that, for most young people, some topics will always remain private from their parents.

Professional practice

The idea that children are sexual beings breaks strong taboos in many cultures and can cause unease among parents and professionals. Teenagers' sexuality can be presented as inherently problematic, with the focus on unwanted pregnancy and STIs causing a blight upon society as a result of 'promiscuity' (Chambers, van Loon and Tincknell 2004).

The only universally accepted sexual activity is that which is seen to take place for reproductive purposes within marriage: this is explicit in most religions and many societies and implicit in others. Sexual deviance is often measured in terms of how far away an activity is from this norm. If children and young people receive negative reactions about their sexuality from adults, they soon learn not to mention sexual matters. Similarly, the sexuality of children and young people is often disregarded by professionals.

Ignoring or avoiding the sexuality of children and young people means missing a whole dimension of important issues and information. Here I return to the two questions introduced at the beginning of this chapter:

1. How is this young person's sexuality affecting his or her behaviour, including what he or she is telling me about symptoms, feelings and relationships?

2. How is the way that I am dealing with this young person going to affect his or her future sexual health, sexual feelings and sexual relationships?

As already indicated, even quite young children may be shy about nakedness and concerned about physical privacy. Children and young people of all ages may fail to disclose symptoms if they fear that disclosure could prompt an unwanted physical examination. Symptoms may be relocated to more 'public' parts of the body and some 'disgusting' symptoms such as discharges not reported at all. Any discussion of menstruation may be experienced as intensely embarrassing, especially with an adult of the opposite sex. Children may feel the need to keep secret their knowledge about sex and reproduction so discussion about future fertility may need to include reassurance and permission to be knowledgeable, together with sufficient explanation to cover gaps and misinformation. Children and young people are often self-conscious about their physical appearance. They may well be ashamed and confused about sexual feelings and embarrassed about romantic attractions, so these may also be kept secret. Their ideas about their future identity as a man or a woman in a relationship, perhaps being a mother or a father, may be too complex to disclose. One of the greatest drivers to secrecy can be if there is any confusion in the child or young person over their sexual orientation or an awareness that they are gay or lesbian. Another is if they have experienced sexual abuse. Any previous experience of professionals being insensitive or disrespectful, especially if confidentiality has not been respected, is also more likely to lead to reluctance to discuss sexual matters.

It follows that services need to pay particular and explicit attention to confidentiality and to the need to reassure potential users of their service about the acceptability of discussing difficult or embarrassing matters. Services need to be provided in a way that demonstrates respect for children and young people and is clear about their needs as individuals distinct from their parents. A primary concern is to obtain sufficient information from the child or young person to be able to provide the best possible care and promote their future sexual well-being.

Children and young people who experience repeated episodes of health interventions or medical examinations, or who need intimate personal care, sometimes feel that their body is not under their own control. They can develop a learned compliance that leaves them more vulnerable to sexual abuse than other children (Westcott and Jones 1999). Sometimes their relationship with their body becomes so dissociated that they do not feel that it is worth looking after. This can lead to poor health choices, including indiscriminate sexual activity. Negative comments from others about weight or physical appearance can contribute to the development of poor body image or even, in more extreme cases, an eating disorder (CMEC [Council of Ministers of Education Canada] 2001). In any discussion of future relationships, care needs to be taken to avoid setting up limiting assumptions that reduce the child or young person's perceptions of the range of experiences and relationships that might be possible for them in the future. Anyone in a caring role should make sure that they do not miss opportunities to give sexual health education and advice as opportunistic approaches can be important complements to more structured programmes of education.

The most important recommendations are the needs for respectfulness, for not being too intrusive and for maintaining the child or young person's dignity and as much privacy as possible in health examinations and consultations. It is important to offer to answer any concerns about sexual and sexual health issues (and to be able to do so comfortably) and to give reassurance about feelings. It is equally important to be honest about the potential effects of any treatment regime on current and future sexual feelings and relationships at the same time as validating and affirming the young person's sexuality. Everyone working with children and young people has a duty to watch out for and report signs of abuse, especially in those children and young people who may find it more difficult to make themselves understood or to recognize that they are being abused.

Conclusion

Children and young people are sexual beings and their developing sexuality is going to affect and be affected by their experience of living with a health condition or treatment that reduces their fertility. Their sexuality and sexual health will similarly affect and be affected by how they are dealt with by the adults around them, including the professionals responsible for their care. The challenge is to ensure that services are provided with sufficient sensitivity and awareness to acknowledge the part that sexuality plays in the life of each individual. The aim is to contribute positively to the child or young person's present and future confidence, identity and capacity for participating in supportive and fulfilling adult sexual relationships.

2

The Views of the Next Generation
An Exploration of Priorities
for Adulthood and the Meaning of
Parenthood Amongst 10–16-year-olds

Claire Fraser, Rachel Balen
and Dorothy Fielding[1]

Introduction

Researchers are increasingly giving young people the opportunity to express opinions on matters that affect them directly (Balen 2000). This view of young people as 'active citizens' (Balen *et al.* 2006) is backed by, for example, the UN Convention on the Rights of the Child (United Nations 1989) and, in the UK, The Children Act (1989) and The Human Rights Act (1998) (Department of Health 2000; Lansdown 1998; Lansdown, Waterson and Baum 1996). Because of our interest in ill health, disability and infertility, we wanted to know more about young people's life ambitions and to find out, in particular, what they think about becoming parents and why adults do and do not have children. We defined this as 'meaning of parenthood'. Some young people will be unable to achieve parenthood because of the fertility-damaging impact of health conditions, disability or treatment. We felt that an understanding of the priorities that children in general have for when they are adults, and of their meaning of parenthood, might be useful to parents and health and welfare professionals. Advice and counselling are needed about the side-effects of health conditions and treatments and any remedial fertility preservation interventions so that informed choices can be made. Such discussions have hitherto been hindered by the lack of research into how young people contemplate parenthood.

Life ambitions

Research has begun to focus on children and young people's priorities for adulthood. Roberts and Sachdev's (1996) UK study examined young people's (12–19 years) social attitudes; amongst the wealth of data generated were findings about ambitions. Fifty-nine per cent of their participants rated their most important life ambition (ranked first or second) as being happy, while 27 per cent wanted to have a family. Good health was important for 24 per cent of the sample, closely followed by having a good job (22%) and being successful at work (20%). Eighteen per cent wanted to be well off and 17 per cent to see the world. These findings were supported by an *Observer*/YouGov poll, which found that almost 66 per cent of 11 to 21-year-olds rated happiness as their most important ambition. Contrary to popular belief, money was much less important to teenagers with only one in six rating it as their greatest priority in life (Summerskill 2002). A UK study by Barry (2001) examining 14 to 27-year-olds' views and experiences of growing up found that a good job was their main aspiration (80 per cent of the sample). Many respondents felt their aspirations were realistic and achievable even though evidence suggested otherwise (many came from areas of high economic deprivation). Raising their own family was the second most important ambition (70%) and for many this was referred to as a way of creating what they themselves had been denied as children: family happiness, stability and consistency.

Meaning of parenthood

Previous research on 'meaning of parenthood' has fallen into two categories:

1. undertaken with adults, largely in relation to infertility and new reproductive technologies

2. undertaken with adolescents, largely in relation to prevention of teenage pregnancy.

Previous research with adults

For the majority of adults there is an expectation and desire to produce children (Edelmann, Humphrey and Owens 1994). Research has suggested that 'meaning of parenthood' is a complex and individual concept with core components (Raphael-Leff 1991) variously identified as biological, psychological, sociological, emotional, interpersonal and socio-cultural/societal. A helpful review of the research in this area has been carried out by Netherwood (1998).

Researchers have also sought to understand the continuing attraction of parenthood. Callan's Australian research (1982, 1983) suggests this may be because virtually all societies are essentially pronatalistic, praising the virtues of parenthood and encouraging reproduction. In British culture, for example, research has shown that there is such a societal expectation to reproduce that those (in particular, women) who either voluntarily or involuntarily do not do so are seen as outside the norm (Blyth and Moore 2001; Greil 1991; Miall 1985; Morell 2000; Woollett and Boyle 2000). The stigma of childlessness, however, is by no means an exclusively female problem. Fathering a child is viewed socially as confirmation of a man's virility (Callan 1982) and a childless man may feel that others doubt his masculinity (Mahlstedt 1985).

Interestingly, the perceived disadvantages of parenthood receive much less coverage in published research. Morse (2000) notes her view that perceived disadvantages may include the inevitable return to traditional roles, with the woman caring for children and being responsible for domestic chores while the man is the primary or only breadwinner; the real or perceived reduction in income and associated financial difficulties; the curtailment of leisure activities; and the prevention of the full experience and expression of an adult relationship because of the presence of a child. An Australian study of voluntarily and involuntarily childless wives' perceptions of motherhood included disruptions to lifestyle, lack of personal time and prevention of opportunities for adult development and learning (Callan 1987).

A review of changing population trends over the past 25 years suggests the need to understand better voluntary childlessness. The number of childless women of 40 years of age in Britain has risen from one in ten in 1980 to one in five in 2000 with women now expected to have an average of 1.7 children each – one of the lowest figures since wartime (Carvel 2000). As Bunting (2004) points out, this trend is not unique to Britain. Although it is commonly assumed that every adult expects and wants to produce children, the prevalence of involuntary childlessness in industrialized societies is around 15–19 per cent (Morse 2000) and research suggests that between 4 per cent (Williams 1987) and 9 per cent (Callan 1987) never seek or want parenthood, preferring instead to pursue careers, enjoy life free from parental responsibilities and commit to relationships without reproduction (Morell 2000; Ussher 2000).

Previous research with adolescents

Previous research about meaning of parenthood amongst non-adults has focused almost exclusively on prevention of teenage pregnancy. Much has focused on females, particularly those who have experienced pregnancy.

In one study, Zabin, Astone and Emerson (1993) examined 'wantedness' (attitudes towards having a baby) amongst 313 inner city Black women under 17 years who presented for pregnancy tests at a US clinic. The questionnaire survey found that 8.5 per cent of them wanted to be pregnant. However, since participants already suspected they were pregnant, their attitudes may have been influenced by impending pregnancy test results. In other American studies, Stevens-Simon et al. (1996) found that 17.5 per cent of 200 pregnant 13–18-year-olds had wanted to become pregnant and Forrest and Singh's (1990) study revealed that 20 per cent of the pregnant 15–19-year-olds surveyed had intended to become pregnant. Rodriquez and Gore (1995) surveyed 341 teenage mothers and found that 31 per cent had intentionally become pregnant.

A study examining prevention of teenage pregnancy in the US (Stevens-Simon, Beach and Klerman 2001) provides a useful meta-analysis of previous research examining why some teenagers are reluctant to actively prevent pregnancy. For example, some thought a pregnancy might improve (or at least not worsen) their relations with family, peers or sexual partners; might help them cope with depression and loneliness; might dispel their concerns about infertility; or might signal their passage into adulthood (Luker 1996; Rainey, Stevens-Simon and Kaplan 1993; Stevens-Simon 1998; Stevens-Simon et al. 1996; Winter 1988). While still concentrating on pregnant or previously pregnant girls, qualitative research has begun to acknowledge that some adolescents view pregnancy and childbearing positively and may desire children (Gordon 1996; Quinlivan and Evans 2000).

It is important to reiterate that the findings of these studies are based on responses from pregnant (or previously pregnant) adolescents and may not therefore reflect the attitudes of never-pregnant adolescents since the unwillingness to acknowledge 'mistakes' may influence participants' responses (Condon, Donovan and Corkindale 2000).

In a recent English study, Bradshaw, Finch and Miles (2005) found that nearly 75 per cent of variation between geographical areas in the teenage conception rate and approximately 50 per cent of variation in the abortion rate could be explained by models of deprivation measured by indicators such as poor education, housing and health, low income and child poverty. Variations in services such as sex education and/or the accessibility of contraceptive advice were thought to provide additional explanations.

While a good deal of research has excluded never-pregnant females, still more has excluded male adolescents. Only three studies could be identified from the last decade and all are American: Marsiglio (1993) surveyed 1880 15–19-year-old males and found that 12 per cent would be pleased if a sexual partner became pregnant. Pleck, Sonnenstein and Leighton (1993) noted that for some young men pregnancy of a sexual partner was seen as a successful 'conquest' and was therefore desired as it endorsed sexual prowess and masculinity. In another study with 350 younger boys (13–14 years), 26 per cent believed they were 'mature enough to be a parent' and up to 15 per cent were noted as having idealized beliefs about the impact of fatherhood on their lives (Robinson *et al.* 1998).

Australian researchers have begun to examine attitudes and beliefs about parenthood (as well as pregnancy and childbirth) among never-pregnant female adolescents and their male peers (Condon *et al.* 2000). This study found that many adolescents (young men in particular) held unrealistic and idealized beliefs about the likely consequences of pregnancy and parenthood. These stemmed from an over-estimation of potential positive aspects and an under-estimation of potential negatives. For example, participants considered that pregnancy would result in greater emotional closeness between partners and increased feelings of happiness. Similarly, parenthood was considered to be linked to closeness, happiness, marital harmony and well-adjusted children. However, participants were unaware of potential negative consequences such as altered lifestyles and difficulties in coping. Condon *et al.* (2000) suggest that many teenage pregnancies are a result of positive, idealized attitudes to pregnancy and parenthood and do not necessarily occur accidentally. Other researchers have identified similar patterns with some participants viewing pregnancy (and hence parenthood) as a 'viable career choice' (Merrick 1995) and press reports have revealed 'extraordinary' requests from teenage girls for IVF treatment, citing pregnancy as their only aspiration in life (Alderson 2004).

Idealized beliefs about parenthood were identified in the 1960s by Le Masters (1970) in a sample of young, White, middle-class Americans. Condon *et al.*'s (2000) research suggests that despite perceived cultural changes since the idealism of the 1960s, present-day adolescent beliefs and romantic ideals transcend social change. This finding may be explained by the fact that adolescents' social cognition appears more susceptible to emotional influence than that of adults and as much as one third of their feelings may be linked to real or fantasized romantic emotions (Larson and Asmussen 1991; Larson and Richards 1994). These findings raise concern, as Condon *et al.* (2000) note. When young people with idealized views actually embark on parenthood, the reality is often met with disillusionment, a potential contributing factor in postnatal depression, domestic violence and child abuse or neglect (Azar and Rohrbeck 1986).

The Study

Our study examined, via the use of a ranking exercise and interview data, children and young people's priorities for adulthood and 'meaning of parenthood'. Our main aims were:

- to explore children's and young people's priorities for adulthood

- to examine where 'having children' fits on their adulthood agendas

- to explore their views about parenthood

- to explore their perceptions about the reasons why some adults have children and others do not.

Method

We used a mixed-methods design with 98 participants. All were pupils from seven schools in the north of England, aged from 10–16 years (mean age 12.8 years). Forty-six (47%) were male and 52 (53%) were female. Ninety-five per cent of the sample were White, two per cent Black Caribbean and two per cent Asian. Local census data confirms that these figures are representative of the local area population. Given the relatively small numbers involved, we did not ask the respondents to declare any disabilities.

All the children and young people completed questionnaires asking them to rank their life ambitions, from a provided list, according to which might be most important for them when they are older. The list of eight ambitions was adapted, with the authors' permission, from those used in an earlier study of young people's social attitudes (Roberts and Sachdev 1996):

- to have good health
- to be in love with someone special
- to have children of my own
- to have good, close friends
- to have a good job
- to have plenty of money
- to own my own home
- to travel and see the world.

Twenty-nine of the males and 31 of the females (approximately ten from each of the six age groups; that is, 10–11, 11–12 etc.) were then randomly selected for individual, semi-structured interviews. These began by asking participants to explain the reasoning behind their ambition rankings. A semi-structured schedule was followed probing their views on reasons why adults do and do not have children.

Findings

Figure 2.1 presents composite percentage rankings for the 98 responses to the ranking exercise. We defined an ambition as 'highly important' if it was first, second or third on their list.

Eighteen per cent (18) ranked the ambition 'to have children of my own' in the top three of their priorities. These responses were then analysed according to age and gender (Figure 2.2) and some differences were observed.

In School Years 6, 7 and 9 this ambition was more important for boys and the reverse was true in School Years 8, 10 and 11. In School Year 7 (11–12 years) boys ranked 'being in love with someone special' and 'having children of their own' significantly higher than did girls. In School Year 8

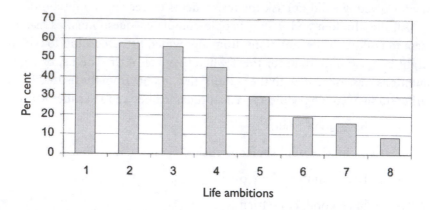

Key: 1 = Friends; 2 = Health; 3 = Love; 4 = Good job; 5 = Money;
6 = Children; 7 = House; 8 = Travel

Figure 2.1 Priorities for adulthood – life ambition rankings (%)

(12–13 years) girls ranked having good friends significantly higher than boys did whereas boys ranked owning their own home higher on their list of priorities than girls. In Year 9 (13–14 years), girls ranked 'having good friends' and 'travelling and seeing the world' significantly higher than did same age boys. Viewing the sample as a whole, girls placed a higher priority than boys on 'travelling and seeing the world'.

A template analysis of the 60 interview transcripts was undertaken (King 1998) and grouped according to whether or not respondents saw parenthood as important. This enabled more detailed exploration of key factors that might have influenced the rankings.

The importance or otherwise of parenthood

Although having children in adult life emerged as something that was ulti-mately very important to many participants, those who ranked it high were more likely to highlight one or more of the following reasons.

Carrying on the human race

Many young people liked the idea of having their own biological child and with it came a sense of 'ownership':

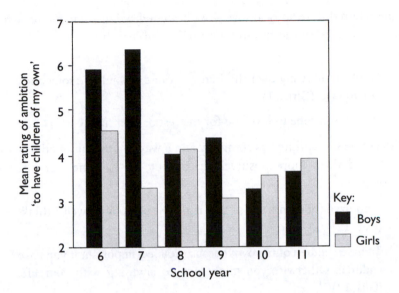

Figure 2.2 Gender and age differences in mean rating of ambition 'to have children of my own' from 2, low importance, to 7, high importance

> ...it's just something that is yours; you can give what you've got to them. (Girl, 16)

For some, this also meant keeping the family (and family name) going; for others this was perceived more widely as continuation of the human race:

> [I want] to have children of my own...to carry on the family name. (Boy, 13)

> [I want] to have children because it is important for me to be able to give something back to the world, that's what we are here for I think. (Girl, 16)

The rewards of loving relationships

Views about love came up frequently. Many saw a close link between a love relationship and having children:

> ...if I am in love with someone special then I can have children of my own. (Boy, 11)

> You've got to be in love to have children so having children comes after love. (Girl, 15)

Some referred to reciprocal love – with a child being someone on whom love could be bestowed through nurturing and/or who could endow their parents with love:

> I'd like to have my own children…because it would be somebody else to love. (Girl, 11)

> It's just someone to love you for the rest of your life. (Girl, 16)

While some saw children as company and a way to prevent loneliness, others viewed them more positively as a route to happiness and feeling complete:

> …to have children because that makes you happy as well I think. (Boy, 12)

> To have children of my own because you feel important if you have children. Otherwise you might not do anything with your life. (Girl, 13)

Some were looking forward to being able to teach their children while others talked of anticipated pride in watching children grow and develop:

> I'd like to have children and watch them grow up. (Boy, 11)

> I want to bring them up and see what they turn out like. (Girl, 14)

The influence of others

Some were influenced in their desire for parenthood by positive accounts from others such as teachers and parents, but this was true only for females:

> I want children of my own because like erm quite a few people have said to me that getting married and having children is the best thing in their life so I'd like to have children of my own…and like [teacher] was saying the other day that the best thing she did was giving birth and just stuff like that. People have just said things and it's made me want to have children when I'm older. (Girl, 11)

It was only females who said their desire for children sprang from experience with children within their own family:

> I'd like to have children…because I think I've grown up with quite a big family and I'm used to like y'know having lots of children around… I've got a niece, she's three, so I look after her a lot. So I've

grown used to y'know having children around so I'd like children of my own to bring up. (Girl, 14)

However, members of both sexes appeared influenced by family members advising them of their potential parenting qualities:

Right, to have my own children…yeah I'd like to have children. My mum said I would be a good dad. (Boy, 14)

Some had arrived at that conclusion for themselves:

I think I would be a good mum. (Girl, 16)

They're so cute…

There were gender differences in seeing babies as desirable in themselves. Some females wanted children because they 'just like babies', often referring to the fact that they are 'cute':

I'd like to have children of my own because I like babies and stuff. My mum's friend has just had a baby and she brought it over for us to have a look at it and she was really cute. (Girl, 11)

I don't want to go into labour or anything like that but I do want children because I think they are sweet. (Girl, 14)

I don't really know why…

Some struggled to find words to explain their strong desire to become parents:

I don't really know why I want to have children of my own but it is something that is important. I couldn't really think of the words to describe it, I just know I want them when I'm older. (Boy, 13)

Then to have children, oh, I can't wait just to have a little one of me or maybe a few of them. I don't know why, it's just to like run about with your kids. (Boy, 16)

Prioritizing other ambitions ahead of parenthood

For some the idea of having children of their own was seen either as not important or as potentially problematic. While the majority indicated that they would probably want children at some stage, there were some who seemed to consider it an unlikely choice. Further analysis from the interviews suggests a mixed picture of 'meaning of parenthood' to this group.

I want to get my ambitions done first

Many indicated that the need to achieve other things in their own lives would take priority over parenthood, at least in early adulthood:

> Yeah. I don't want children like straight away. I want to get my ambitions done first… I want to settle into and then get used to my like own life like cos I'll be going out into the big wide world… And I want to get used to all that and then settle down. (Girl, 14)

> I would like to have a family of my own but I'd probably concentrate on getting my own life sorted out first, education wise, going to college and then if someone comes along, settle down and have children of my own. (Boy, 16)

Too young to think about it…

Some felt they were too young to think about parenthood yet and it appeared to have little meaning for them:

> It would be nice to have children but you don't think about it as a major thing at this age. (Girl, 11)

> …it will probably change, it is just what I think now [don't want children]…when I get older though I will probably want to have children. (Boy, 12)

Others saw age as important in a different way – that having children was not a priority in their life ambitions because parenting was something that was only appropriate at certain ages:

> It's something I never thought about when I was younger, I used to think I would want to be at least 35 before I got married but now I want to be young so I can enjoy it. My dad is older so he never got to go out and do stuff with me so I want to be young when I have kids so I get to go out and play football with them. (Boy, 16)

Some participants seemed unaware of age limitations on women's fertility status:

> Well I'm not bothered because you can have them whenever you like…if you want to you can and if you don't you don't need to have them. (Girl, 11)

Importance of being in an adult relationship

For some in this group, being in a relationship was more of a priority than having children, though some linked this to parenthood by seeing relationship stability as a necessary precursor to having children:

> I wouldn't want to have children at the beginning because my Mum and Dad always say to me you don't want to have children before you get settled down or anything, you have children when you've settled down with someone special. (Girl, 12)

Need for financial security

This group were more likely to talk about the potential financial burden of children and the need for financial security before contemplating parenthood:

> You need to have your job and house and money first before you can do that [have children]. (Boy, 13)

> No, I don't know [why having children is low down on list]. I think want to be able to give them a good life so I want to have plenty of money first so I can bring them up properly. (Girl, 15)

Lack of desire to have children...

Among those who did not appear to want to have children at all, some arrived at this decision because of prior experience with younger children, such as siblings and cousins:

> I'm not that bothered about having children... I don't think I will have the patience... I've got a cousin that always comes every Monday and she drives me mad. (Girl, 11)

> I don't know, I'll have to see. I'm not really good with children, well little children when I play with them and all that, they always seem to get on my nerves you see. (Boy, 14)

Participants across the age sample had clear thoughts about the burdens that children may impose:

> I like children, little babies, but they are very noisy and tire you out. (Girl, 11)

> But I reckon they [children] would be hassle so that is why it's last. Like you've got to stop working if you've got a full-time job, it just

turns your life plan on its head. Like my sister, she had a good job and now she has had a baby she sits at home all day, that's her life, it's boring. I don't really want one because of that. (Boy, 15)

Discussion

The children and young people in our study indicated that their most important ambition was to have good friends. In School Years 8 and 9 (12–13 and 13–14 years) this was more important for girls than for boys. The second most important ambition was the desire to have good health. Third was to be in love with someone special and in School Year 7 this was more important for boys than for girls. The desire to have children was much less important, appearing low down on the overall rankings and considered to be only marginally more important than owning a house and travelling/seeing the world.

The overall importance of friends is not surprising given the age of the sample. Previous research has documented the importance of peer group relationships during middle childhood and adolescence and this is often particularly true for girls (see Cottrell 1996). The importance of the desire for good health is also supported by research that has documented the health concerns of young people (Ackard and Neumark-Sztainer 2001) and their health information seeking behaviours (Borzekowski and Rickert 2001). The relative importance of being in love with someone special in adulthood is to be expected as it has been noted that young people's conceptions of love are consistent with adults' conceptions regardless of whether or not they have experience of romantic love (Connolly *et al.* 1999). However, the finding that this ambition was significantly more important for boys than girls in Year 7 was unexpected. Gender stereotyping generates the expectation that boys would not routinely place a high value on so-called 'feminine' emotions such as love. Our finding questions gender stereotypes about what is important for boys and girls at different ages.

Although the ranking exercise was slightly adapted for inclusion in this study, the findings on priorities for adulthood do not support the earlier findings of Roberts and Sachdev (1996). In our study having good health was seen as considerably more important and having children considerably less important. It is possible that such differences in the ranking of ambitions have occurred because of age-group differences in the two samples.

Those in Roberts and Sachdev's (1996) study were 12–19-years-old and the inclusion of young adults may have increased the relative importance of childbearing since this is more likely to be on the agendas of 17–19-year-olds than it is for 10–11-year-olds.

Although 'having children of my own' was seen by our sample as less important than other ambitions, clear age and gender differences emerged in the rankings given, although statistically significant gender differences were only observed amongst Year 7 pupils. Marked age difference fluctuations were noted as opposed to a consistent pattern of either increasing or decreasing importance. It is unclear exactly why these fluctuations have emerged and further research is indicated. The onset of puberty may provide a partial explanation as fewer extreme gender differences are observed post-Year 8. The transition from primary to secondary school and increased interaction with the opposite sex post-puberty may also be a possible explanation. In addition, it may be that the steady increase in the importance of the desire for children for participants during Years 10 and 11 may be due to increasing awareness of societal expectations to reproduce in adulthood.

It is clear that while some children and young people may have idealized beliefs about parenthood, others are able to comprehend the limitations and difficulties that children might bring. The potential problems of parenthood highlighted by the children in this sample are consistent with previous research with adults (Callan 1983, 1987; Ussher 2000).

Age was another theme in meaning of parenthood. The notion of being too young to think about having children was discussed by younger participants and many older participants had clear thoughts about the age at which they would want their own children. This indicates an understanding of the notion of planned life events. One finding from our study is that while not all children and young people were *currently* thinking about having children of their own, some expressed their awareness that their views would change as they got older. Many indicated that they expected to be parents at some point in their adulthood and that they could anticipate how it might feel to be unable to have children (see Chapter 3).

The gender and age differences observed in participants' ranking of ambitions and priorities for adulthood indicate that we do need to be wary of adopting stereotypical ideas about what may be important for boys and for girls at different ages. Contrary to popular belief, boys may place a high priority on future parenthood. This finding contradicts previous research, which has suggested that boys do not grow up thinking of themselves as future fathers (Mahlstedt 1985). The message is that time and care must be taken by adults in ascertaining individual children's current and future ambitions for adulthood.

Note

1 We would like to thank The Candlelighters Trust for funding the research cited in this and the following chapter. We would also like to thank Dr Ian Lewis, the children and schools who took part in the study and the local Education Authority who supported the work.

3

Children and Young People's Understanding of Infertility

*Rachel Balen, Claire Fraser
and Dorothy Fielding*

Introduction

Our interest in children's understanding of infertility, its causes and treatment alternatives available, stemmed in part from the experience one of us
had of being the parent of a child diagnosed with a form of cancer and in
part from random conversations held with young paediatric oncology
patients during the course of a participant observation research project
some years ago (Balen 2000). Both experiences led us to wonder how far
adults recognize and understand the knowledge base and insights held by
children and young people. We realized that current levels of knowledge
and understanding amongst children about (in)fertility, its impact and the
techniques available to 'treat' it could only be speculated upon because of a
lack of research in this area. Indeed our literature searches revealed no such
research activity. Heke and Alexander (1995) focused on young adults and a
major study of children's sexual thinking (Goldman and Goldman 1982)
failed to address the issue at all. The authors of this latter study noted
Clautour and Moore's (1969) earlier finding that the majority of boys and
girls looked forward to marrying and having children, but their own study
equated 'not having babies' only with a knowledge of contraception.
Equally, their vocabulary-testing methodology included an understanding
of pregnancy, conception and contraception but not of (in)fertility.

We were aware of the importance of informed understanding amongst adults who live with, care for, work with, support and/or treat those children and young people who are born with or acquire health conditions or disability in their childhood or teenage years that may have an adverse effect on their fertility. Such experiences in the lives of children and young people may not only have an impact on the way they see themselves and how they view their lives, but may also affect their sense of difference from peers, a group who set norms and attitudes about such issues as relationships, sexuality and what it means to be adult.

We could not assume that the concept of infertility is unknown to children and young people: as avid watchers of British TV 'soaps', also much watched by children and young people, we knew that episodes have featured a husband with a low sperm count (*Eastenders*, BBC1 1998), a surrogacy arrangement (*Brookside*, Channel 4 1998) and a couple undergoing IVF treatment (*Brookside*, Channel 4 2001).

The Study

Our study focused on responses from a population of children and young people in mainstream education rather than specifically from those receiving medical treatment for illness, living with a health condition or disability or receiving special education. This sample was chosen in order to provide some benchmark information since discussions about infertility and possible fertility preservation options sometimes have to be entered into at a time of diagnosis; that is, before any psychological, physical, emotional and cognitive changes that treatment and its effects may bring about (Eiser 1993). The fieldwork was located in seven schools in the north of England and involved 98 pupils from School Years 6–11 (10–16 years of age).

In researching understandings and perspectives we were keen to explore these questions:

- Are children and young people aware that some people cannot have children?

- Do they have any knowledge of possible causes and treatments?

- What are the sources of the above knowledge?

- Are they aware of the possible emotional consequences of being unable to have children?

- What ideas do they have about how people who can't have children might feel?

In order to inform the development of appropriate psycho-social interventions for those diagnosed with cancer or other relevant populations, we were also keen to find out:

- how they think a child or young person being offered fertility preservation might feel

- what they think they might want to know

- who they think they might want to speak to

- whether they understand the vocabulary used by adults in health settings.

Methodology

We approached all the primary (ages 5–11 years) and secondary schools (ages 11–16 or 18 years) within the Local Education Authority (LEA). The seven schools, one primary and six secondary, which both responded positively and could meet with us within our timeframe, were located in a range of inner city, suburban and semi-rural locations. Their pupils were representative of those within the LEA with regard to gender, parental socio-economic status and ethnicity. In the secondary schools each year group was divided into several classes. In each of these schools we invited all pupils within one of the relevant year group classes to participate in the research. A total of 98 completed a questionnaire designed to collect demographic data and explore their priorities for adulthood. This was achieved by asking participants to rank a series of ambitions (see Chapter 2). Sixty were then randomly selected and invited to take part in individual semi-structured interviews. The sample was made up as shown in Table 3.1.

The interviewer probed the participants' views on reasons why adults do and do not have children and their knowledge of infertility and fertility preservation. Research interventions are not neutral processes: we wanted to ensure that we did not introduce any new knowledge (for example, making a previously unaware child or young person aware of the notion of

Table 3.1 Individual interview participants

School Year	Male	Female	Sub-total
Year 6 (10–11 years of age)	5	5	10
Year 7 (11–12 years of age)	5	5	10
Year 8 (12–13 years of age)	5	5	10
Year 9 (13–14 years of age)	6	6	12
Year 10 (14–15 years of age)	3	5	8
Year 11 (15–16 years of age)	5	5	10
Total	29	31	60

infertility) and were mindful of the comments from concerned school parent-governors who had given permission for our pilot study:

> Don't they have enough to cope with as it is, without worrying about whether or not they may be infertile?

> Sex education is enough of a 'hot potato' as it is, this venture could just complicate matters further.

For these reasons the interview schedule had a potential pre-determined cut-off point. Those who demonstrated no prior knowledge of infertility finished the interview here and moved on to the vocabulary section (see below). Those who demonstrated a prior knowledge of infertility were presented with two vignettes. The first concerned an infertile couple and participants were asked questions to ascertain their knowledge of treatment and treatment prospects. They were also asked to comment on the possible emotional reactions the couple may be experiencing and who they might prefer to speak to. The second vignette concerned a child patient in hospital (matched in terms of gender and age to the respondent) who was to undergo treatment that might damage fertility. They were asked to comment on what the hypothetical child's emotional reaction might be, who they might want to talk to and what they might want to know. Questions were also asked to determine whether respondents had any knowledge of fertility preservation and, if so, the sources of their knowledge. Finally, all were asked to consider a vocabulary list containing medical and fertility-related words and explain what they thought the words meant and where they thought they had first heard them.

In any research, participants should be clear from the outset that they are free to withdraw at any time and this is particularly important when conducting research with children and young people. We explained to those taking part in the interviews that they did not have to respond to every question if they did not wish to do so. To aid this process, coloured cards were used to allow them to retain control of the interview. Each participant was given a red and yellow card before the start of the interview and advised that the yellow card could be used to skip a question and the red could be used to end the interview. (We chose these colours as we thought that most would be familiar with the yellow 'booking' and red 'sending off' cards used in football!) We felt the cards were an important non-verbal tool, as the thought of telling an adult researcher that they did not wish to continue might have been a daunting prospect. In the event, the red card was used by one Year 6 boy to terminate an interview and the yellow card was used by two Year 6 boys to move on to the next question. Interviews were tape-recorded, transcribed and analysed using Template Analysis (King 1994).

Findings

Analysis of the 60 transcripts focused on:

- knowledge of infertility
- understanding of vocabulary
- awareness of infertility issues
- sources of advice and support for those experiencing involuntary childlessness
- possible tests and treatments for infertility
- emotional consequences
- fertility preservation options

- sources of knowledge

- issues of consent.

Knowledge of infertility

We defined 'knowledge' as an awareness of childlessness and the inability to have children. We found that 30 of the 31 females interviewed had this knowledge; only one of the youngest (Year 6) girls was unaware. Amongst the males, the results were slightly more variable. Four of the five in each of Years 7 and 11 had this knowledge as did three of the five in Year 8. Four of the six males in Year 9 were aware, as were two of the three in Year 10 and two of the five in the youngest group, Year 6. Prior knowledge was therefore present in 19 of the 29 males.

Understanding of vocabulary

All 60 participants were shown the following words: *anaesthetic; operation; surgeon; consultant; paediatrician; cells; ovary; sperm; egg; genes; organs; Fallopian tubes; conception; sterility; infertility; preservation; donor; gametes; gonads; IVF.* These were chosen following perusal of child cancer patient information leaflets and websites, assisted conception unit leaflets, children's storybooks and dictionaries. The LEA sex education policy and British Government guidance on sex and relationships education were also consulted to ensure that words presented were already covered in the school curriculum for all the year groups in the study. Analysis indicated some inaccuracies and con-fusions in understandings. Although participants might have indicated that they did understand a particular word, their definitions were sometimes inaccurate. For example, a 15–16-year-old might indicate to us that they understood the word 'sperm' but they were unable to accurately define it (for example, 'the man's part of a baby' – female aged 15). Others confused 'conception' with 'contraception'.

Understanding of vocabulary came from five main sources – the media (TV, films, magazines), school/books, friends, family and own experience (visits to doctors, dentists, hospitals). The media and family were the most frequently cited.

Awareness of infertility issues

The 30 females and 19 males who had shown that they knew about the notion of infertility were then shown the two vignettes described above. Their responses reveal their insights into the following:

1. causes of infertility

2. sources of advice and support for those experiencing involuntary childlessness

3. possible tests and treatments for infertility

4. emotional consequences

5. fertility preservation options

6. sources of their own knowledge.

Causes of infertility

Responses about causes of infertility ranged from the vague to the specific and included biological problems caused by defect, disease or accidental damage; sexual preference; choice; and 'bad luck'. Infertility was seen as something that could be present at birth or happen later:

> No, there are biological problems with adults... I don't really know that much but I just know that some people can't have children because they have something wrong with them. I think they might be born that way. (Boy, 13)

> I know someone who had a cyst on her ovary and so they're infertile now. (Girl, 16)

> ...or like they've had a crash and it's done something to their ovaries. Libby (in *Neighbours*) broke up with her boyfriend over that because Drew wanted a baby but she couldn't have one... Yes, like if she's been in a crash. (Boy, 11)

Although all spoke of adults *choosing* not to become parents, only one child referred to this choice resulting in a man's *inability* to have children and there was no mention of female sterilization.

> Well, they might have had, oh, what's it called, like vasos, the man, to stop him having children, is it a vasectomy? The man might have that. (Girl, 12)

What some were explicit about was that fertility is randomly and perhaps unfairly distributed:

> Not all are able. Some are able but just don't want to, but some aren't able to have children but do want to. (Boy, 13)

> Well some people, they have problems don't they, and some people have bad luck. (Girl, 15)

A significant feature of responses was that although participants demonstrated awareness that some adults are not able to have children, they were hazy or confused in their understanding about possible causes of this and about the relationship between fertility and sexuality:

> ...not everyone does. Like transsexuals, I'm not sure but I don't think they can have them. (Boy, 13)

> Some people can't have them cos like they don't, y'know some people just can't have them...just like, they're just infertile aren't they or there is something wrong with their organs and stuff or they could be gay or lesbians and stuff so not unless y'know... (Girl, 14)

Sources of advice and support for those experiencing involuntary childlessness

The first vignette featured an adult couple unable to conceive a child. Participants were asked what they thought the couple might do next and where they might turn for help. Responses included consulting local or specialist doctors, seeing psychiatrists and specialist counsellors and talking to family and friends:

> ...I think they would rather go to their GP rather than a hospital or clinic because if they go to their GP they would probably know him for a number of years. Like I've known mine since I lived in that area. I think they would maybe feel more comfortable with their friends but the doctor needs to help them with medical stuff. (Girl, 16)

One of the common elements of many responses was embarrassment:

> They might go to a counsellor, a specialist in this sort of problem. They might discuss it with their family. But they might keep it to themselves because they might be embarrassed about it. (Girl, 12)

> There might be a GP that comes round to them or a clinic, they might go there. I wouldn't [feel comfortable talking to the doctor]

talking about my bits. I'd want to talk to a man about it, not a nurse. (Boy, 11)

Some showed great maturity and insight:

> Erm, go and see a doctor to get more information, to see if he knows why, if it is a medical reason. They might talk to close members of the family to see if they know why before or they might go straight to the doctor… It depends on what type of relationship they've got with the rest of the family. If it's a very close one they probably won't mind talking to the rest of the family but if they sort of distance themselves from the rest of the family or are just not on good terms with them they will probably prefer the doctor. (Boy, 13)

Responses during discussion of the second vignette, concerning a hypothetical child cancer patient undergoing treatment that may impair fertility, revealed a similar theme but with stronger emphasis on gender and family relationships:

> Probably if he had an older brother then he would want to talk to him but I don't think an older sister, his Dad maybe or he could want to talk to a male doctor. I don't think, he might want to talk to his mum about it, I think more likely a male. (Boy, 12)

> Her friends or a woman doctor. Because I wouldn't feel very comfortable talking to a man about this sort of thing and erm a counsellor… Not my parents, I know they love me and they're very understanding but I don't really like talking to them about serious decisions or serious things about my life. I don't know. My parents never spoke to me about sex or anything like that… (Girl, 14)

When participants were asked what they might want to know, their answers ranged from specifics to muddle:

> He'd like to keep asking questions, like about what the percentages are of whether he will not be able to have babies or whether he will. And he will want to find out like how bad his actual disease is. Find out the history of the tests and of the operation what they are going to do on him, find out how many kids, how many people have been able to have babies when they are older and how many haven't… Also if the people who are doing it have ever performed it before and what have been the outcomes of what they've done before and he can like be asking like his mum if she would have married his dad if he'd not been able to have babies and stuff like that. Just be asking

people, just like trying to find out if he was guaranteed to not be able to have babies or not. (Boy, 11)

She'd probably have loads of questions running around her head but when she came to ask them they might be all mixed up. (Girl, 12)

Possible tests and treatments for infertility

Many had only a vague understanding with much uncertainty and confusion evident:

Erm, they would probably just go and see the doctor to see if they could have some tests done to see if anything was wrong... I don't know [what tests] really, I'm really not sure. They can get treatment for it if they really wanted to have children... They maybe, they might be able to have an operation to do something that meant that they could or something like that, I don't really know exactly what... I don't know [if the treatments work], I don't even know if they are really possible, I'm just guessing. (Girl, 12)

Others revealed a slightly clearer understanding:

Or check for tests and things to see if there was anything wrong with them both... Well just check the woman's womb to make sure she is OK and the man too, check that he is OK in that department [laughter]. Erm, they could have treatment, like IVF...well, if the woman can't have children then they get donor eggs and things and put them together with the man and then implant it in the woman. Or it can be the other way round if it is the man with the problem, they get donor sperm and do it like that. I saw it on TV. (Girl, 14)

Not all responses were wholly accurate:

They do like sperm counts on the man to see if he is fertile or not, I'm not sure what the lady's test is called, oh I think it is a smear test... I'm not sure whether they can treat it. (Boy, 16)

Emotional consequences

Some participants demonstrated insight into adult emotions when asked how a couple who had been unable to have a baby might feel. Their responses captured feelings of sadness, anger and anxiety:

[They would feel] disappointed, not so much at the fact that they can't have children but at each other as if it's their own fault…and erm anger that so many other people can have children by accident or just straight away almost and they've had to try and still not had one… (Boy, 13)

Some felt the couple would gain solace from the knowledge that they could have a child by another means, revealing their own rather simplistic views of what are in fact complex processes with uncertain outcomes:

They might be a bit upset if they're not able but they could always adopt so it wouldn't mean that they couldn't have children at all. They would probably be upset and sad too. (Girl, 11)

Other responses revealed an awareness of societal expectations:

They might be depressed; always on a downer; feeling like they aren't human because they can't have kids… (Girl, 14)

The depth of some of the insights displayed by children as young as 11 or 12 years old was striking:

Erm, just really, really upset, confused because they might not know why they can't have a child, they might not have told them so they just don't know and that will make them sad. Really emotional because sometimes it's mainly women who find it harder to cope with because they can't bear children like their mother did, so they might find it really emotional. Angry towards the other partner because if say the female can have a child and her partner can't, no matter how much she loves him she may feel angry that she can't have a child with him. In fact the only way she can have a child is not with him and she would always know that it is not his child. But if they love each other enough they will stay together and work it out. (Girl, 12)

They might be feeling pretty sad because they know they can't have a baby that will have their genes and that…they won't like be feeling really down because they still know that they can have a baby by donor sperm or surrogate mother or adoption but they will, they'll feel like that if they do get a baby they'll feel like it's not actually theirs, it's sort of theirs but it's someone else's as well. And it will, they won't know, like if say they had a surrogate mother, the woman won't know what it's like to actually have a baby inside her and carry it and feel it kick and everything like that so they'll miss out on all the emotion of childbirth and everything like that. (Boy, 11)

Responses to the vignette in which a child was being offered medical treatment that might impair fertility also revealed insightful thinking:

Well, I think she might not be able to take it all in. She might think oh well I'm only young…it might not hit her until she is older and she has decided that she does want children and she might think will anyone want me, will anyone want to be with me, will I get a partner because they might think I want to settle down and have a family and I can't because I can't have children. Erm, it might, I think if I got told it would really upset me because I do want to have children when I'm older but it might not really click until I'm older but she would be really upset. (Girl, 12)

I think he would be kacking himself and wanting to go to that sperm bank thing and he would be like proper angry…because if you like choose to get rid of the illness you can't have a kid and everyone else would have kids and you couldn't so you would be the loner. And your partner might leave you because you can't have kids so you'd be a loner again. (Boy, 15)

Fertility preservation options

Knowledge of fertility preservation options was probed during discussions about the situation facing the child patient in the second vignette. Some responses contained elements of greater accuracy than others:

Well, they do an operation on you where they take an egg out of your ovary and they take like a test tube and they freeze it until like you want a baby and then they take some sperm and put it with it and try and fertilize the egg and then when it is fertilized I think, I'm not sure, I think they put it back inside you, yeah I think they put it back inside you so that your womb can start developing to help you have a baby. (Girl, 14)

Could they like, could they like take his sperm and put it back into him after the operation again? (Boy, 11)

One 13-year-old boy's knowledge included an awareness of wider implications:

> They could erm, what's it called, it's like a sperm bank, have it in storage for when he's older in case he does cos he's religious, whatever religion, or his parents' wishes, but they could do that. But he might definitely decide that he does not want children, he might not like children or he might be scared. (Boy, 13)

Several females were aware of the possibility of freezing eggs, but some were less than clear about the process:

> Well is it if you haven't started your periods yet then your eggs don't get I don't know, grow or anything, I don't know. (Girl, 14)

Sources of their own knowledge

Much of their knowledge was gained from the media, for example television, films and magazines:

> Erm, TV and things like that I think... *Casualty, Peak Practice*, I don't think we've done it in school. (Girl, 13)

Some used television watching experiences as a springboard for discussions with parents:

> *Coronation Street.* I don't know if you watch it. Hayley and Roy, they can't have children. Libby on *Neighbours*. Yeah, probably something I saw on TV and then asked my mum. Whenever I see something on TV that I think is strange I always ask my mum to explain. (Boy, 11)

Others recounted personal family experiences:

> Probably because my auntie had to adopt some children because I asked my mum why and she said that she couldn't have children so we talked a bit about that. That was quite a while ago. (Boy, 12)

Some were clear that their knowledge came from school while others had acquired knowledge in more informal ways:

> ...in Biology. (Boy, 16)

> ...probably my old school, in my junior school. I remember I was with my friend James and we were looking through books and stuff cos we had to like learn about them things so we were looking through... so we were there reading through this massive book and it said not all people can have children and I thought eh? So we were like asking our class teacher why can't and then she was explaining

to us why. So I think that's how I probably knew about it. I was like oh, I hope I'm not one of them. (Boy, 14)

I don't know. It's just like your friends know so you know. (Boy, 11)

Consent

Many had clear views about who should consent to fertility preservation treatment, views that were not unanimously shared:

Her [the child in the vignette] definitely. If it was me and my mum didn't want me to have it I would be really frustrated and annoyed that she has the right to answer for me when it is my life and my future family so it should definitely be Sally. (Girl, 16)

Her mum, because she is the parent so she decided what happens to her daughter. (Girl, 16)

Him because it's his life that's ahead of him so it should be his choice provided that he is mature enough to think about it. But if he is not mature it should be his parents. (Boy, 15)

Other responses revealed more general thoughts about the power of adults over children:

Normally…the parents try to persuade the child to have the treatment and I guess normally the 12-year-old wouldn't get a say in it, it's not just the doctors that ignore children. (Girl, 12)

I think they ought to treat everyone the same but normally in hospitals they treat 12-year-olds like children and 16-year-olds like adults but if a 12-year-old and a 16-year-old have the same condition then they should hear the same things but normally they don't. Sixteen-year-olds get spoken to more professionally and the doctors only speak to the parents when you are 12 but it is the child who needs to know. (Girl, 12)

Discussion

This study aimed to explore the current level of awareness and knowledge about infertility amongst children and young people. The responses raise a range of issues for consideration.

It is clear from the responses to the two vignettes that adults need to be wary of adopting stereotypical notions about children and young people's understandings of the impact of (in)fertility on human emotions and rela-tionships. Both males and females revealed equally insightful thinking at times and equally confused or hazy knowledge at others. Nor was insightful or clear thinking restricted to the older age group – some of these were far less knowledgeable and informed than younger children.

Not all children and young people *currently* think about having children of their own in adulthood. However, many indicated that parenthood is cer-tainly something they expect to achieve in their twenties or thirties. It is clear that some are already aware of the societal expectation of reproduction and can anticipate how it may feel to have this 'right' removed from them (see Chapter 2). Many interviewees referred to adoption as an easy solution to involuntary childlessness and were clearly unaware of the difficulties and delays involved.

Social researchers are increasingly acknowledging the importance of understanding children and young people's perspectives as these may differ from and be better developed than accounts based on what adults think children think. (See, for example, Alderson 2000; Borland *et al.* 1998.) The sophisticated and sensitive responses of children as young as 11 or 12 in this study reinforce the need for adults not to underestimate children and young people's capacities. At the same time, the inconsistent and sometimes confused knowledge base revealed by participants lends support to the need for health and welfare practitioners to provide 'able instruction' (Vygotsky 1962) to enhance children and young people's understanding when necessary. However, the information and explanations offered, partic-ularly to those who may be sick and frightened, may need to be revisited over time in order to maximize the chances of being heard, understood and assimilated. Communication between adult professional and young patient will also need to include clarification of the words being used. In our study, many participants indicated that they knew and understood the meaning of words but in reality this understanding was muddled or inaccurate. This has important implications for health professionals communicating with chil-dren and young people. Careful exploration is necessary to ensure that they really do understand the terminology discussed since they may give the impression that they have a greater understanding than is the case.

Responses to the vignettes revealed a wide range of individual differ-ences. Some were clear that if they were in the situation depicted, they themselves would want to talk to doctors; others would prefer parents to speak on their behalf. Those working with young patients will need to explore and understand an individual's preferences. As Lockwood, Cooklin and Ramsden (2004) point out:

> an individual child's view of the concept of consent will be influenced not only by their age and maturity but also by the nature and degree of anxiety associated with, and previous experience of, the illness, and therefore the degree with which a child may expect and/or wish to hand over control to his or her parents. (p.201)

A child or young person's expectation of (non-)participation in such decisions will also, as these authors suggest, be influenced by the cultural traditions of the family involved.

At some regional paediatric oncology centres, fertility preservation is currently being offered to young patients (Crawshaw *et al.* 2003; Glaser, Wilkey and Greenberg 2000; Wallace 2000). The need to understand what children do and do not understand about infertility and medical terminology is central to this practice, as is an understanding of the emotional consequences such treatment may bring for them (Broome and Allegretti 2001).

The findings from our study may prove useful in informing the consultations between health and welfare personnel, children and young people and their parents and in the design of psycho-social interventions that are age appropriate and relevant to individual situations. As Green, Galvin and Horne (2003) have noted, the timing and level of such consultations have hitherto been based on intuition since no previous studies have examined children and young people's understanding in this area. Research (Cook 1999; Dixon-Woods, Young and Heney 1999) continues to stress the importance of involving children and young people in medical decision-making. Stacy Nicholson and Byrne (1993, p.3399) noted that 'Even if they do not ask...information should be part of the informed consent process' and their involvement may help to 'attenuate the stresses actually experienced' (Lansky, List and Ritter-Sterr 1986, p.531).

Finally, as Wallace and Thompson (2003) have commented:

> Open discussion is...often potentially therapeutic for the vulnerable family facing treatment... Discussion of fertility issues at the time of diagnosis provides the family with the reassurance that...the team believe in a future when these issues will become important. (p.493)

Part Two

Medical, Scientific, Legal and Ethical Aspects of Compromised Fertility in Adolescence and Early Adulthood

4.

Health Conditions and Treatments Affecting Fertility in Childhood and Teenage Years

Adam Balen and Adam Glaser

Introduction

Fertility, defined as the capacity to conceive, is an essential component of an individual's health. Even though some adults will make their own decision not to have a family, the potential to make this personal choice is an important component of their autonomy. The practical implications of infertility will not become apparent until the age of sexual maturity and in most cases many years later in adult life. However, many of the causes of fertility impairment may be congenital or acquired during childhood and adolescence. This chapter will outline some of these.

In the management of young people with fertility problems one must be sensitive to the specific needs of the adolescent who may be confronted with issues relating to sexual function, sexual identity, endocrinology and fertility. Adolescents may have difficulty raising issues of sexual function or reproductive health difficulties with their doctors (Malus *et al.* 1987) and may present with complaints of minor symptoms rather than their primary concerns (Patton 1999). Effective history-taking from an adolescent requires particular skills and sensitivities. When dealing with pre-existing conditions or treatments during childhood, the young person's parent is often present and embarrassment about discussing menstruation, anatomy and sexual intercourse may mean that problems are either not discussed or otherwise only with parental prompting. Effective services must recognize these patterns and plan accordingly.

Puberty

Puberty and adolescence are recognized as involving marked endocrine changes, which regulate growth and sexual development. Normal pubertal development is known to be centrally driven and dependent upon appropriate gonadotrophin[1] and growth hormone (GH) secretion in addition to normal functioning of the hypothalamic-pituitary-gonadal axis. Onset of puberty usually occurs between the ages of 8 and 13.5 years in girls and 9 and 15 years in boys. The mechanisms that control the precise timing of onset, however, are still not clearly understood but are influenced by many factors including general health, nutrition, exercise, genetic influences and socio-economic conditions.

Nutrition and body weight play an important role in pubertal development. In females, chronic disease, malnutrition, severe dieting in an attempt to conform to a perceived 'ideal' of slimness and high levels of physical activity can delay menarche (onset of menstruation). There has been much interest in the actions of the hormone leptin, which may potentially have a role in signalling the hormonal control of pubertal development (Mantzoros, Flier and Rogol 1997). Intense exercise, such as long-distance running, ballet, rowing, long-distance cycling and gymnastics, is associated with delayed menarche in young girls and with amenorrhoea (absence of periods) in older women (Frisch *et al.* 1981). These 'endurance' sports are associated with lower bodyweight and percentage fat.

There is no doubt that while many menstrual cycles are initially anovulatory[2] some may be ovulatory, often with a long follicular phase (Venturoli *et al.* 1986). Early menarche is associated with early onset of ovulatory cycles. When menarche occurs below 12 years, 50 per cent of cycles are ovulatory in the first year and virtually all by the fifth year. By contrast, it takes 8–12 years for all cycles to be ovulatory in girls with later onset of menarche (Vikho and Apter 1984). This has important clinical implications for advising adolescents and their parents or carers on the 'normality' of their menstrual pattern relative to their age at menarche.

Precocious puberty

Precocious onset of puberty is defined as occurring younger than two standard deviations (SDs) before the average age; that is, earlier than eight years old in females and earlier than nine years in males. Thus, in many individuals, early onset of puberty merely represents one end of the normal distribution. However, a number of pathological conditions may prematurely activate the GnRH-LH/FSH (hypothalamo-pituitary secretory unit) axis, resulting in the precocious onset of puberty (see Table 4.1). Investigation and treatment of precocious puberty should always be by a paediatric endocrinologist.

Table 4.1 Causes of precocious puberty

Gonadotrophin dependent ('true' or 'central' precocious puberty)	Idiopathic (family history, overweight/obese)
	Intra-cranial lesions (tumours, hydrocephalus,[a] irradiation, trauma)
	Gonadotrophin-secreting tumours
	Hypothyroidism[b]
Variants	Premature thelarche[c] (and thelarche variant)
	Adrenarche[d]
Gonadotrophin independent	Congenital Adrenal Hyperplasia (CAH)[e]
	Sex steroid-secreting tumours (adrenal or ovarian)
	McCune Albright Syndrome[f]
	Exogenous oestrogen ingestion/administration

Notes

a Condition where fluid accumulates in the brain.

b Abnormally low activity of the thyroid gland.

c First stage of breast development.

d Increased secretion of adrenal androgens, usually just before age eight.

e Inherited condition affecting adrenal glands. Females are born with masculine appearing external genitals but internal female sex organs. Males appear normal at birth.

f Genetic disease affecting bones and skin pigmentation, which also causes hormonal problems and premature puberty.

Delayed puberty

Delayed puberty is defined as absence of onset of puberty by more than two SDs later than the average age; that is, later than 14 years in females and later than 16 years in males. Delayed puberty may be idiopathic/familial or due to a number of general conditions resulting in undernutrition. Absence of puberty may also be due to gonadal failure (elevated gonadotrophin levels), or impairment of gonadotrophin secretion (see Table 4.2).

Table 4.2 Causes of delayed puberty

General	Constitutional delay of growth and puberty
	Malabsorption (e.g. coeliac disease, inflammatory bowel disease)
	Underweight (due to severe dieting/anorexia nervosa, over-exercise)
	Other chronic disease
Gonadal failure (hypergonadotrophic[b] hypogonadism)[c]	Turner Syndrome[a]
	Polyglandular autoimmune syndromes
	Post-malignancy (following chemotherapy/radiotherapy)
Gonadotrophin deficiency	Congenital hypogonadotrophic hypogonadism (anosmia – lack of ability to smell)
	Hypothalamic/pituitary lesions (tumours, post-radiotherapy)
	Rare inactivating mutations of genes encoding LH, FSH or their receptors

Notes

a Congenital condition of females associated with a defect or absence of an X-chromosome, characterized by short stature, sexual underdevelopment etc.

b Involving increased production or excretion of gonadotrophic hormones.

c Inadequate functioning of testes or ovaries.

Management depends on cause. Following exclusion of other diagnoses, many patients with constitutional delay are happy to await spontaneous pubertal development. However, severe delay in pubertal onset may be a risk factor for decreased bone mineral density and osteoporosis. In children with hypergonadotrophic hypogonadism, puberty may be induced from any age. However, for others, such as girls with Turner Syndrome, delay in induction to around 14 years old possibly permits maximal response to growth hormone therapy.

Menstrual cycle abnormalities

Amenorrhoea

Amenorrhoea (the absence of menstruation) may be temporary or permanent (usually of at least six months' duration). It is best classified according to its aetiology, or site of origin, and can be subdivided into:

- disorders of the hypothalamic-pituitary-ovarian-uterine axis
- generalized systemic disease.

The failure to menstruate by the age of 16 in the presence of normal secondary sexual development, or 14 in the absence of secondary sexual characteristics, warrants investigation. This distinction helps to differentiate reproductive tract anomalies from gonadal quiescence and gonadal failure. Primary amenorrhoea may be a result of congenital abnormalities in the development of ovaries, genital tract or external genitalia or a disturbance of the normal endocrinological events of puberty (see Table 4.3).

Overall it is estimated that endocrine disorders account for approximately 40 per cent of the causes of primary amenorrhoea. The remaining 60 per cent result from developmental abnormalities. All of the causes of secondary amenorrhoea may be found to cause primary amenorrhoea (see Table 4.4).

Investigation of amenorrhoea, whether primary or secondary, will usually be as set out in Table 4.5 and treatment determined as appropriate.

Oligomenorrhoea

Oligomenorrhoea may be defined as menses occurring less frequently than every 35 days. The commonest cause of oligomenorrhoea is polycystic ovary syndrome (PCOS). Other causes include either temporary disturbances of menstrual cycle control or the development of one or more of the causes of secondary amenorrhoea.

Table 4.3 Classification of primary amenorrhoea

Disorders of the hypothalamic-pituitary-ovarian-uterine axis

Uterine/vaginal causes	Müllerian agenesis[a] (e.g. Rokitansky Syndrome)
Ovarian causes	Polycystic ovary syndrome[b] (PCOS)
	Premature ovarian failure (genetic, e.g. Turner Syndrome, or acquired following pelvic radiation or chemotherapy)
Hypothalamic causes (hypogonadotrophic[c] hypogonadism)	Weight loss
	Intense exercise (e.g. ballerinas)
	Idiopathic
Delayed puberty	Constitutional delay or secondary (see text)
Pituitary causes	Hyperprolactinaemia[d]
	Hypopituitarism[e]
Causes of hypothalamic/pituitary damage (hypogonadism)	Tumours (craniopharyngiomas, gliomas, germinomas, dermoid cysts)
	Cranial irradiation
	Head injuries (rare in young girls)
Systemic causes	Chronic debilitating illness
	Weight loss
	Endocrine disorders (e.g. thyroid disease, Cushing's Syndrome)[f]

Notes

a Müllerian ducts fail to develop and a uterus will not be present in a female.

b Cysts in the ovary interfere with ovulation and menstruation.

c Reduced production or excretion of gonadotrophic hormones.

d Too high levels of prolactin in the blood.

e Low levels of pituitary hormones.

f Hormonal disorders caused by exposure to high levels of cortisol.

Table 4.4 Classification of secondary amenorrhoea

Disorders of the hypothalamic-pituitary-ovarian-uterine axis

Uterine/vaginal causes	Asherman's Syndrome[a]
	Cervical stenosis[b]
Ovarian causes	Polycystic ovary syndrome (PCOS)
	Premature ovarian failure (genetic, autoimmune, infective, radio/chemotherapy)
Hypothalamic causes (hypogonadotrophic hypogonadism)	Weight loss
	Exercise
	Chronic illness
	Psychological distress
	Idiopathic
Pituitary causes	Hyperprolactinaemia
	Hypopituitarism
	Sheehan's Syndrome[c]
Causes of hypothalamic/pituitary damage (hypogonadism)	Tumours (e.g. craniopharyngiomas)
	Cranial irradiation
	Head injuries
	Sarcoidosis[d]
	Tuberculosis
Systemic causes	Chronic debilitating illness
	Weight loss
	Endocrine disorders (e.g. thyroid disease, Cushing's Syndrome)

Notes

a Intrauterine adhesions as a result, typically, of scar formation after uterine surgery.

b Narrowing of the spinal canal.

c May occur in a woman who has severe uterine haemorrhage during childbirth, resulting in tissue death in the pituitary gland.

d Involves inflammation that produces tiny lumps of cells which may clump and affect how an organ works.

Table 4.5 Investigation of amenorrhoea

Physical examination	Note body mass index, pubertal development, stigmata of PCOS and other endocrine disease
Endocrine assessment	Pregnancy test if suspected
	FSH, LH
	Prolactin
	Thyroid function tests
	Testosterone (if stigmata of PCOS)
	Further endocrinology only if above do not provide diagnosis
Pelvic imaging	Ultrasound: morphology of ovaries and endometrial thickness (for oestrogenization)
	MRI if suggestion of complex developmental problem
Pituitary/hypothalamic imaging	MRI if indicated
Bone mineral densitometry	If at risk of osteoporosis
Karyotype[a]	If premature ovarian failure

Note

a An organized profile of a person's chromosomes.

Polycystic ovary syndrome

The polycystic ovary syndrome (PCOS) is the commonest endocrine disturbance affecting females. It may occur as a syndrome by itself or it may be associated with other health conditions or disabilities. The presence of enlarged ovaries with multiple (at least 12) small cysts (2–9 mm) and a hypervascularized[3] androgen[4]-secreting stroma[5] are associated with signs of androgen excess (hirsutism, alopecia, acne), obesity and menstrual cycle disturbance (amenorrhoea or oligomenorrhoea) (Balen et al. 1995). There is considerable heterogeneity of symptoms and signs amongst women with PCOS and for an individual these may change over time, as may her needs (e.g. cycle control versus fertility). Furthermore, polycystic ovaries may be seen without clinical signs of the syndrome, which may then become expressed over time. In 2003 a new definition of PCOS was agreed internationally; this requires the presence of two out of the following three criteria, with the exclusion of other aetiologies (Fauser *et al.* 2004):

1. oligo- and/or anovulation

2. hyperandrogenism (clinical and/or biochemical)

3. polycystic ovaries.

Ovarian dysfunction leads to the main signs and symptoms of the PCOS and the ovary is influenced by external factors, in particular the gonado-trophins and insulin, which are themselves dependent upon both genetic and environmental influences. Approximately 20–33 per cent of women of reproductive age will have polycystic ovaries on ultrasound scan (Michelmore *et al.* 2001; Polson *et al.* 1988); while perhaps 75–80 per cent of these will have symptoms consistent with the diagnosis of PCOS. There are long-term risks of developing diabetes and cardiovascular disease (reviewed by Rajkowha *et al.* 2000). The long-term risk of endometrial hyperplasia[6] and endometrial carcinoma due to chronic anovulation and unopposed oestro-gen has long been recognized; similarly there may be an increased risk of breast carcinoma (Balen 2001). For women with PCOS who experience amenorrhoea or oligomenorrhoea, it is advisable to induce artificial with-drawal bleeds to prevent endometrial hyperplasia. Indeed, women with PCOS should shed their endometrium at least every three months. For those with oligo-/amenorrhoea who do not wish to use cyclical hormone therapy we recommend an ultrasound scan to measure endometrial thickness and morphology every 6–12 months (depending upon menstrual history).

The PCOS is a heterogeneous condition, with not all signs and symp-toms existing concomitantly in an individual. The clinical management of a young woman with PCOS should be focused on her individual problems. Obesity worsens both symptomatology and the endocrine profile and so obese women (BMI > 30 kg/m^2) should therefore be encouraged to lose weight. They should also have a test of glucose tolerance (e.g. two-hour GTT). There is evidence that females from South Asia have a greater degree of insulin resistance than White Caucasian females and so assessment of glucose tolerance should be performed at a BMI of ≥ 25 kg/m^2 (Wijeyaratne *et al.* 2002).

Hyperandrogenism and hirsutism are the most distressing symptoms for young women. Optimally treatment combines cosmetic and medical therapies. Medical regimens stop further progression of hirsutism and slow the rate of hair growth. However, drug therapies may take six to nine months or longer before any benefit is perceived and so physical treatments including laser, electrolysis, waxing and bleaching may be helpful while waiting for medical treatments to work. Medical therapy is aimed at slowing the rate of hair growth while cosmetic treatments attempt to remove existing hair.

The simplest way to control the menstrual cycle in women with PCOS is the use of a low dose combined oral contraceptive preparation (COCP). This will result in an artificial cycle and regular shedding of the endometrium. It is also important once again to encourage weight loss. As women with PCOS are thought to be at increased risk of cardiovascular disease, a 'lipid friendly' combined contraceptive pill should be used. Insulin sensitizing agents, such as metformin, are becoming increasingly popular in the management of PCOS as they act directly at the pathogenesis of the syndrome and help correct both metabolic and endocrine problems. Early studies suggest an improvement in reproductive function and menstrual cycle regulation and there may be benefits to health of long-term use, including deferring the onset of Type 2 diabetes, although large prospective studies are required (Balen 2004).

While fertility is not usually a concern of adolescent girls with PCOS, their mothers or fathers will often ask about potential fertility if their daughters have erratic menstrual cycles. The key advice concerns diet and body weight, as being overweight in the long term both reduces spontaneous fertility and the chance of a response to ovulation-inducing drugs if required (Balen 2004).

Hypothalamo-pituitary dysfunction

Secondary hypogonadism results from deficiency of luteinizing hormone (LH) and follicular stimulating hormone (FSH). The primary deficiency arises from the pituitary or hypothalamus. Hypopituitarism may be idiopathic or secondary to tumours of, or adjacent to, the hypothalamic-pituitary axis. In childhood and adolescence, these include craniopharyngiomas, germ cell tumours and adenomas. Radiotherapy to the central nervous system for the treatment of brain tumours or leukaemia may result in acquired failure of the hypothalamic-pituitary axis with secondary infertility.

Isolated deficiency of gonadotrophin-releasing hormone (GnRH) affects 1 in 10,000 males and 1 in 50,000 females. It may be part of Kallmann Syndrome, which is associated with anosmia (lack of sense of smell) and is due to deletion of the single gene, Kalig-1, which results in abnormal neuronal migration during fetal life (Bick *et al.* 1992; Skakkebaek, Giwercman and de Krester 1994).

Infertility secondary to cancer and cytotoxic treatments

Childhood cancer is rare – the risk for an individual child developing cancer in the United Kingdom before the age of 15 years is 1 in 500. Seventy-three per cent of patients are still alive five years after diagnosis (Toms 2004). Both radiotherapy and chemotherapy may directly damage the ovary or testis, while tumours and radiation to the brain may affect the hypothalamo-pituitary axis (see above). The extent of resulting infertility is unclear as:

- new cancer therapies are constantly developing that may prove more damaging or less damaging to the reproductive system than those currently used

- survival and therefore the potential for reproductive recovery is further prolonged.

Additionally, new assisted reproductive techniques are developing (Multi-disciplinary Working Group 2003).

Currently it is thought that 15 per cent of survivors will have a high risk of early and irreversible gonadal failure, while others may have a lower risk of compromised reproductive capacity (Wallace *et al.* 2001). Males appear to be more susceptible to sub-fertility following chemotherapy than females, while some females may be at risk of premature menopause.

Cytotoxic therapies, including cyclophosphamide, are used to treat non-malignant conditions in childhood and adolescence including some chronic renal and rheumatoid conditions. Consequently, survivors of these conditions may be at risk of impaired fertility, although lower doses of chemotherapeutic agents are usually used in the management of these disorders.

Abnormalities of female genital tract and intersex disorders

Congenital absence of the vagina

Mayer-Rokitansky-Kuster-Hauser Syndrome (MRKH or Rokitansky Syndrome) occurs in 1:5000 female births and may be associated with renal tract anomalies (15–40%) or anomalies of the skeletal system (10–20%).

Girls have spontaneous development of secondary sexual characteristics as ovarian tissue is present and functions normally. The external genitalia have a normal appearance but the vagina is short and blind ending. Hormone treatment is not required as ovarian oestrogen output is normal and ovulation will take place. However, the only route to biological parenthood will be through using a surrogate mother following ovarian stimulation and oocyte (unfertilized egg cell) retrieval. This will clearly require careful discussion with all concerned.

The vaginal dimple can vary in length from just a slight depression between the labia to up to 5–6 cm. Vaginal dilators, made of plastic or glass, are used to stretch the vaginal skin and the patient is encouraged to apply pressure for 15 minutes twice daily with successive sizes of dilator. An adequately sized vagina is usually formed by six months but this may take longer and long-term use of dilators may be required, depending upon the frequency of sexual intercourse. A number of surgical approaches have been employed to create a neo-vagina, although are rarely required.

Diagnosis is often not made until puberty or sometimes not until commencement of sexual activity. It can usually be made without the need for a laparoscopy. Sometimes, however, an ultrasound scan will reveal the presence of a uterine remnant (anlagan), which is usually small and hardly ever of sufficient size to function normally. If there is active endometrial tissue within the uterine anlagan, the patient may experience cyclical pain and the anlagan should be excised (usually laparoscopically).

Fusion abnormalities of the vagina

Longitudinal fusion abnormalities

These may lead to a complete septum (dividing wall) that may be associated with two complete uterine horns with two cervices or a partial septum causing a unilateral obstruction. Excision is required both to prevent retention of uterine secretions and to permit sexual intercourse.

Transverse fusion abnormalities

These usually present with primary amenorrhoea and require careful assessment before surgery. The commonest problem is an imperforate hymen in which a cyclical lower abdominal pain combines with a visible haematocolpos[7] and a bulging purple/blue hymen with menstrual secretions stretching the thin hymen. The surgery required is a simple incision, which should be performed when the diagnosis is made to prevent too big a build up of menstrual blood, which may lead to a haematometra[8] and consequent increased risk of endometriosis (secondary to retrograde menstruation). A transverse vaginal septum, due to failure of fusion or canalization between the Müllerian tubercle and sino-vaginal bulb, may present like an imperforate hymen but is associated with a pink bulge at the introitus as the septum is thicker than the hymen. Great care must be taken during surgery to prevent annular constriction rings and the procedure should only be performed in dedicated centres by experienced surgeons. When there is a transverse septum it has been found to be high in 46 per cent of patients, in the middle of the vagina in 40 per cent and low in the remaining 14 per cent. It is the patients in the last two groups who have higher pregnancy rates after surgery.

Müllerian/uterine anomalies

Uterine anomalies occur in between 3 and 10 per cent of the fertile female population and are often discovered by chance during coincidental investigations for infertility. They have usefully been classified by the American Society for Reproductive Medicine into five groups. Women with uterine anomalies are usually asymptomatic, unless there is obstruction to menstrual flow, when cyclical pain may be experienced. While infertility per se is rarely caused by uterine anomalies, they may be associated with endometriosis if there is retrograde menstruation secondary to obstruction. Furthermore, recurrent miscarriage may be experienced by some women with uterine malformations.

Surgery is reserved for those cases where there is obstruction, for example the removal of a rudimentary uterine horn or excision of a vaginal septum. The excision of a uterine septum has been shown to improve pregnancy outcome and should be performed by an experienced hysteroscopist. On the other hand, metroplasty[9] (Strassman procedure) of the horns of a bicornuate (having two horns) uterus is currently seldom performed as its benefit has been questioned.

Abnormalities of male genital tract

Bilateral castration and anorchia[10] (incidence of 1 in 20,000 males) are rare causes of absent testicular tissue. Other rare anatomical causes of male infertility include agenesis (absence) of the epididymis or other parts of the ductal system including the vas deferens. The latter is found in most males with cystic fibrosis (CF). The majority of males found to have isolated bilateral agenesis of the vas deferens without any other signs of CF have been found to be carriers of a point mutation in the CF gene. In these individuals, genetic counselling is indicated (Editorial, *Lancet* 1992).

Genetic causes of male infertility

Males with Klinefelter Syndrome (also known as 47,XXY or XXY after an additional X chromosome these individuals have; incidence of 1 in 1000 males), some of whom also have learning disabilities, invariably have azoospermia.[11] Prior to puberty the seminiferous tubules (which make up the bulk of the testis) develop normally but during puberty a massive destruction of the seminiferous epithelium (tissue lining of the tubules) occurs.

XYY males (47,XYY; incidence of 1 in 1000) have varying degrees of spermatogenic impairment and may be fertile. Autosomal[12] chromosomal translocations result in a heterogeneous pattern of fertility impairment. Micro-deletions in this region (Yq11) may result in disturbed spermatogenesis or azoospermia and probably account for 10–15 per cent of idiopathic azoospermia and severe oligospermia,[13] with higher prevalence in more severe testiculopathies, such as Sertoli-only Syndrome (Ferlin *et al.* 1999; Kun, Inglis and Sharkey 1993).

Undescended testis

The undescended testis (cryptorchidism) is associated with infertility as well as tumours and torsion (abnormal twisting of the testis). Cryptorchidism is bilateral in 30 per cent of cases and infertility occurs in these individuals. Interestingly, where there is a contralateral testis (the descended testis), this may have impaired spermatogenesis, suggesting that some people with maldescended testes have a congenital defect of the germ cell population (Giwercman *et al.* 1989).

Cryptorchidism is found in 0.7 per cent of males after one year of age. The incidence increases with prematurity and is found in 100 per cent of 28-week gestation neonates. After the first year of life, spontaneous descent does not occur. To minimize the risk of malignancy, torsion and infertility, treatment before two years of age is indicated.

Varicocele

The pampiniform venous plexus (a vein) at the back of the testis is dilated in this condition. Varicocele[14] is rare in children under ten years of age although occurs in 15 per cent of adult males (there are no figures available for adolescents). Subfertility may result through decreased spermatogenesis and sperm motility. Surgical ligation of the internal spermatic vein may result in increase in testicular size and improved fertility.

Intersex disorders

Intersex conditions consist of a 'blending' or mix of the internal and external physical features usually classified as male or female (Creighton and Minto 2001). Prevalence is difficult to ascertain due to different definitions of the condition, although range between 0.1 and 2.0 per cent (Blackless *et al.* 2000). These are very rare conditions and must be managed in centres familiar with them. A multi-disciplinary team (MDT) that includes paediatric surgeons, urologists (often paediatric and adult), plastic surgeons, endocrinologists, specialist nurses, social workers, psychologists and also gynaecologists is required. The MDT usually makes a decision during infancy, in conjunction with the parents, as to whether the child should be raised as a boy or girl. Gender assignment is primarily determined by how the individual will develop and how it is thought that they may prefer to live post-puberty when they become sexually active. Guidelines have been proposed on this (Diamond and Sigmundson 1997). Individuals with mixed gonadal dysgenesis (faulty development) or true hermaphrodites are usually assigned gender according to the size of the phallus or extent of labia/scrotum fusion.

Ambiguous genitalia

Disorders of sexual development may result in ambiguous genitalia or anomalies of the internal genital tract and may be due to genetic defects, abnormalities of steroidogenesis and dysynchrony during organogenesis (formation of the organ[s]). Age of presentation will depend upon the degree of dysfunction caused. The incidence of genital ambiguity that results in the child's sex being uncertain is 1 in 4500, while some degree of male undervirilization or female virilization may be present in up to 2 per cent of live births (Ogilvy-Stuart and Brain 2004).

Genital ambiguity can be due to undervirilization of an XY individual, virilization of an XX individual or, most rarely, due to true herma-phroditism. In the latter condition, ovarian tissue with primary follicles and testicular tissue with seminiferous tubules are present, either in separate gonads or within ovotestes.

XX females can be virilized due to increased fetal androgen production (including Congenital Adrenal Hyperplasia), fetal gonadal androgen pro-duction, transplacental passage of androgen, dysmorphic syndromes, bisexual gonads (hermaphroditism).

XY males can be undervirilized due to: testicular malfunction, de-creased fetal androgen biosynthesis, end-organ unresponsiveness, maternal oestrogens, dysmorphic syndromes.

Androgen Insensitivity Syndrome (AIS)

Complete Androgen Insensitivity Syndrome (CAIS, formerly known as testicular feminization syndrome – a term that is no longer favoured) is an example of undervirilization of an individual with 46XY karyotype. Patients usually present as phenotypically normal girls but have absent pubic and axillary hair in the presence of normal breast development. In this condition, while testes are present, there is an insensitivity to secreted androgens because of abnormalities in the androgen receptor. The inci-dence is approximately 1:60,000 'male' births. Anti-Müllerian factors prevent the development of internal Müllerian structures and the Wolffian structures also fail to develop because of the insensitivity to testosterone, although the external genitalia appear female. In about 10 per cent the defect is incomplete (PAIS – Partial Androgen Insensitivity Syndrome) and the external genitalia may be ambiguous at birth with labio-scrotal fusion. Virilization may sometimes occur before puberty.

After puberty, gonadal tissue should be removed to prevent malignant transformation (dysgerminoma), which otherwise occurs in about 5 per cent of cases. Exogenous oestrogen should then be prescribed: cyclical treatment is not required because the uterus is absent. The syndrome may be diag-nosed in infancy if a testis is found in either the labia or an inguinal hernia,[15] in which case both testes should be removed at this time because of the potential risk of malignancy. Some cases, however, only present at puberty with primary amenorrhoea. Removal of abdominal/inguinal testes should then be performed.

Congenital Adrenal Hyperplasia (CAH)

This condition can cause virilization of XX females or undervirilization of XY males. Females are likely to show signs of female pseudohermaphroditism[16] with signs of masculinization at birth, clitoromegally (enlarged clitoris, simulating a penis), varying degrees of fusion of the labial-scrotal folds and, sometimes, a urethral fistula. Surgery may be undertaken with great care during the neonatal period and may be required again during adolescence. As with all surgery for intersex disorders, the precise timing is open to debate as is the degree to which the patient – rather than her parents and physicians – is involved in the decision-making process.

Females with CAH invariably have polycystic ovaries and a tendency to express a PCOS-like condition. One of the best indicators of good therapeutic control of CAH, and hence avoidance of infertility, is a regular menstrual cycle. Males appear normal at birth and develop premature physical sexual development over the first five years of life.

Summary

Fertility may be affected by a wide range of either congenital or acquired conditions in childhood and adolescence. While the consequences of these conditions may not become functionally important until adulthood, the fertility consequences must not be ignored as early intervention may minimize the extent of reduction in fertility capacity and may help individuals come to terms with opportunities available to them in later years.

Notes

1 Gonadotrophin is a hormone capable of producing gonadal (sex organ, i.e. ovary or testicle) growth and function.
2 Not properly developing and releasing a mature egg every month.
3 Having a large number of blood vessels.
4 Hormone that controls the development and maintenance of masculine characteristics.
5 The connective supportive framework of a cell, tissue or organ.
6 Benign condition where the lining of the uterus (endometrium) grows too much.
7 Accumulation of menstrual blood in the vagina.
8 Accumulation of blood in the uterus.
9 Surgical procedure used to reshape the uterus and uterine cavity.
10 Absence of both testes at birth.
11 No sperm present in the ejaculate.

12 Pertaining to any chromosome that is not a sex chromosome.
13 Having too few sperm.
14 Mass of enlarged veins that develops in the spermatic cord.
15 Hernia in the groin.
16 Congenital abnormality where external genitalia of a male or female resemble those of the opposite sex.

5

Fertility Preservation Methods and Treatments for Females

Helen Picton

Introduction

Fertility preservation techniques are relevant to young girls and adolescents for many reasons. While these technologies can be used to preserve the eggs and ovaries of young trauma patients, or girls with a familiar history of early menopause, to date they have been predominantly aimed at safeguarding the fertility of young women and girls who are diagnosed with cancer and treated when they are too young to have either started or completed their families. High-dose chemotherapy regimes are also being used for an increasing number of non-malignant conditions such as autoimmune diseases and thalassaemias. While the ovaries of young patients can be protected from the destructive effects of such treatments, either surgically or pharmacologically, recent advances in cryobiology mean that it is now also possible to freeze-store the eggs and ovarian tissues from young patients. For adolescent girls, secondary oocytes (unfertilized egg cells) can be cryopreserved (preserved by cooling sub-zero temperatures) by either slow freezing or ultra rapid freezing (vitrification) techniques. However, the efficiency of this procedure is unacceptably low. The only option available to preserve the fertility of pre-pubertal girls is the cryopreservation of immature primordial oocytes *in situ* within fragments of ovarian cortex. Once the patient is in remission and wishes to start her family, the frozen-thawed tissue can be autografted back into the body in its usual (orthoptic) or different (heterotopic) position to restore natural fertility. However, if there is any risk of reintroducing cancer cells in the graft, a safer alternative is to grow folli-cles and oocytes contained within the tissue to maturity *in vitro*. The efficiency and safety of this approach needs validation prior to clinical implementation.

Background

There are a number of incidences where young patients may wish to protect and/or preserve their future fertility. Fertility preservation may, for example, be advocated in girls and adolescents undergoing surgical interventions where the ovaries must be removed as a consequence of abdominal trauma. For adolescents and young women who have a familial history of premature ovarian failure, it may be foolhardy to delay child-bearing (Conway 2001; Davis *et al.* 2000). These patients may elect to preserve their oocytes or ovar-ian tissue to prolong their reproductive lifespan. Girls with Turner Syndrome have a very high risk of premature menopause or, in the most severe cases, they may be permanently sterile. The former group of individ-uals may elect to cryopreserve their ovarian tissue during their pre-pubertal or early teenage years before their ovarian reserve is completely lost and menopause ensues (Hreinsson *et al.* 2002; Saenger *et al.* 2001).

The overwhelming application of fertility preservation techniques to date is to those patients who are at risk of temporarily or permanently losing their fertility as a result of cancer treatment. For this group of patients the documented late effects of pelvic irradiation, with or without treatment with alkylating chemotherapy agents,[1] include reduced pregnancy rates in young women and a high risk of partial or total ovarian failure (Meirow 2000; Meirow and Nugent 2001). While the preservation of fertility in young cancer patients forms the main focus of this review, the biology sur-rounding the onset of early menopause and the methods used to preserve and restore the fertility of cancer patients can be applied to any young patient, regardless of diagnosis, who is at risk of premature loss of their ovarian function.

Irrespective of the diagnosis of a young patient it is clear that, in the ovary, the number of oocytes is limited, it is fixed since fetal life, and it can-not be regenerated (Faddy *et al.* 1992). When the reserve of the earliest staged primordial follicles and the primordial oocytes they contain has been exhausted (on average this would occur naturally in women around age 50) menopause occurs. Thus, surgical removal of ovarian tissue or exposure to radiation or alkylating agents and platinum compounds will permanently and prematurely deplete the ovarian reserve and so render young patients of any age temporarily or even permanently infertile (Bath *et al.* 2001; Meirow 2000; Wallace, Thomson and Kelsey 2003). Furthermore, it appears that the extent of gonadal damage induced by irradiation or chemotherapy depends on the patient's gender, age at the time of treatment, radiation dose and fractionation schedule and the total dose and nature of chemotherapy delivered (Grundy *et al.* 2001a). Partial or total loss of fertility is particularly relevant to young girls who, in the event of ovarian failure, are faced with the prospect of lifelong hormone replacement therapy – a regime that is not, in itself, risk free. Until such a time as medical treatments can be directly targeted to malignant cells, health care professionals are faced with the challenge of not only devising improved treatment strategies that protect the individual's well-being, but also of developing and implementing protocols that will protect and/or conserve the fertility of these young patients.

The options for preserving the fertility of young female patients range from no medical intervention at all to the use of invasive procedures to harvest tissues or isolated cells from the ovaries. Each method has its own advantages, disadvantages and risks. The approaches that can be used to protect the fertility of girls and adolescents can be divided into three broad categories: prediction of ovarian damage; protection of the ovaries; and preservation of oocytes (Table 5.1).

Prediction of ovarian damage

The ability to measure the likely toxic impact of chemotherapy and radiation exposure regimes on the ovaries of pre- and post-pubertal girls would enable us to predict how such treatments will affect the future reproductive lifespan and fertility of these individuals (Singh, Davies and Chatterjee 2005). Tests of ovarian damage must assess the number of primordial follicles present in the ovary (the ovarian reserve) rather than the number of more advanced growing follicles and mature oocytes, as the later stages of follicle and oocyte development are less likely to survive the treatment. Hundreds of thousands of primordial follicles are present in the ovaries of young patients (Gougeon, Echochard and Thalabard 1994); of these follicles only 400–500 would ovulate during the reproductive lifespan of a woman. The usual fate of the vast majority of the follicles present in the ovary is therefore degeneration through a process termed apoptosis (Gosden and Spears 1997). There is, therefore, a vast redundancy in the ovarian reserve and a significant proportion of the follicles and oocytes present in a

**Table 5.1 Treatment options for preservation
of fertility in young, female cancer patients**

Treatment options	Methodology	Suitability/Applicability
Prediction of the impact of chemo- and radiotherapy on the lifespan of the ovary	In vitro exposure diagnostic study	All patients[a]
	Exposure studies in model species	All patients
	Measurement of ovarian reserve	All patients
Reduction of the risk of ovarian damage	Ovarian transposition	Adults and adolescents
	GnRH agonist or antagonist co-treatment	All patients
	Oral contraceptive pill	Adults and adolescents
Preservation and restoration of fertility	Cryopreservation of embryos after IVF	Adults
	Egg donation	Adults
	Cryopreservation of MII oocytes	Adults and adolescents
	Cryopreservation of GV oocytes	All patients
	Cryopreservation of ovarian tissue	All patients

Note

a All patients = adults, adolescents, and pre-pubertal girls.

young ovary can be lost as a consequence of treatments without unduly compromising the future fertility of the individual. In support of this concept, there are numerous reports of young women who suffer a transient loss of reproductive cyclicity following cancer treatment before their hormonal and reproductive cycles are re-established and their natural fertility is restored (Meirow 2000). The ability to assess accurately the ovarian reserve in these individuals, both before and after their cancer treatment, would provide these patients with reassurance that their cancer treatment has not induced a premature menopause.

Ovarian follicle reserve can be assessed in a number of ways but much debate exists as to the accuracy and reliability of the different methods

(Gülekli *et al.* 1999). Histological assessment of surgically recovered ovarian tissue has been used to assess the density of primordial follicles in the human ovary (de Bruin *et al.* 2002, 2004). This approach relies on the fixed tissue sample being representative of the whole of the ovary, which unfortunately is frequently not the case. Alternatively, ultrasound measurement of ovarian volume has been proposed as an indicator of ovarian function in women post-cancer treatment (Sharara and McClamrock 1999). Similarly, measurement of the ovarian hormone Inhibin B, which is secreted into the peripheral circulation by the granulosa cells of small antral follicles, has been suggested as an index of ovarian function (Hall, Welt and Cramer 1999; McLachlan *et al.* 1986). While the measurement of ovarian volume and Inhibin B levels are useful, both of these techniques measure the number of advanced antral follicles in the ovary and thus only provide a snapshot of ovarian function at the time of the assay. Neither of these methods provides long-term insight into the reproductive lifespan of the individual as they do not measure the number of primordial follicles left in the ovary. A far more informative approach, which has been successfully applied to the prediction of ovarian reserve in adult cancer survivors, is the measurement of the systemic level of Anti-Müllerian Hormone (AMH) (Bath *et al.* 2003). The concentration of AMH in the blood accurately predicts the reproductive lifespan as AMH is synthesized and secreted only by primordial follicles.

Protecting the ovaries

Evidence suggests that it is possible to shield vulnerable organs such as the ovaries from the damaging effects of cancer treatments. The ovaries can be surgically moved out of the direct path of radiation exposure. Ovarian transposition can be to an alternative location in the abdomen or to a heterotopic site such as the forearm (Oktay and Karlikaya 2000). While this ovarian transposition has been used in adults with limited success, it is not a long-term solution for the preservation of fertility in younger patients.

An alternative protective approach, which is suitable for girls, is based on the idea that the pre-pubertal ovary is relatively quiescent and can be pharmacologically protected from the cytotoxic effects of medical therapies that destroy rapidly dividing cells. The drugs that can be used to limit the gonadal toxicity of otherwise successful treatments include gonadotrophin-releasing hormone (GnRH) agonists and antagonists. These synthetic hormones are based on the endogenous brain peptide GnRH and are routinely used in reproductive medicine to reversibly shut down ovarian function and induce a hypogonadotrophic[2] state. In the context of shielding the ovary of a young patient, the GnRH analogue would be administered before the start of chemo- or radiotherapy to suppress the release of the follicle stimulating hormone (FSH) and luteinizing hormone (LH) from the brain (Bath *et al.* 2001). FSH and LH normally drive cell division and promote growth in ovarian follicles. If the cells in the follicle are actively dividing, they are more vulnerable to the cytotoxic damage by chemo- or radiotherapy treatments. Administration of drugs such as GnRH agonists during treatment would therefore be expected to protect the ovaries by inhibiting the later stages of follicle growth. In support of this idea, Ataya *et al.* (1995) demonstrated in primates that GnRH-agonist co-treatment protected the Rhesus monkey from cyclophosphamide (an alkylating agent) induced ovarian damage. These findings are supported by several clinical studies. For example, co-treatment with GnRH agonist during chemotherapy resulted in premature ovarian failure in only 2.3 per cent of patients compared with 58 per cent in the group treated with chemotherapy only (Blumenfeld *et al.* 1996). GnRH agonist administration to adolescents during chemotherapy has also been shown to confer some degree of protection on the ovary (Pereyra Pacheco *et al.* 2001). While these studies are encouraging, conflicting evidence raises doubts as to the benefit of this approach (Gosden *et al.* 1997; Howell and Shalet 2001) and for the most part the data remain unconvincing.

Programmed cell death by apoptosis has been identified as the mechanism responsible for both the loss of oocytes that occurs during the normal process of oogenesis (the process by which mature ova are produced in the ovary) (Gosden and Spears 1997) and for oocyte loss induced by anti-cancer therapies (Morita and Tilly 2000). Preliminary evidence has implicated sphingosine[3]-based lipid signalling molecules such as ceramide and sphingosine-1-phosphate (SIP) as key mediators of cellular growth, differentiation and apoptosis in postnatal ovaries (Morita *et al.* 2000). This observation has opened new avenues for protecting the ovaries of patients from possible side-effect damage. Treatment of mouse ovaries *in vitro* with SIP resisted the apoptosis induced by anti-cancer therapy, whereas *in vivo* injection of SIP into the ovarian bursa of mice completely prevented radiation-induced oocyte loss (Morita *et al.* 2000). Further research is required to explore the potential protective effect of small lipid molecule therapy on the ovaries of young patients.

Preservation of oocytes

The current options available to preserve the fertility of young patients, irrespective of their diagnoses, are limited. The methods used include assisted reproductive techniques such as *in vitro* fertilization (IVF), which enable collection and freeze storage of embryos before myeloablative[4] cancer treatment (Atkinson *et al.* 1994). However, assisted reproduction is costly and stressful, carries no guarantee of success, may create 'orphan embryos' if the woman dies and requires that the patient has a male partner. A further disadvantage of assisted conception is that sick patients must undergo an extended protocol of four to nine weeks of ovarian monitoring, down regulation (whereby drugs are used to block the natural mechanism that releases eggs) and drug stimulation to produce sufficient mature oocytes for IVF, embryo production and freezing. Consequently, very few recently diagnosed cancer patients, for example, have sufficient time to go through an IVF cycle before they start their cancer treatment. Furthermore, in the case of steroid-related cancers, the ovarian hyperstimulation required for assisted reproduction may be contraindicated. Perhaps most importantly, embryo cryopreservation is not an option for young girls.

An ethically acceptable alternative to embryo freezing, which is suitable for young patients of all diagnoses, is the cryopreservation of oocytes. Two practices can be used to freeze-store oocytes; these are:

1. cryopreservation of fully grown secondary oocytes at either the germinal vesicle (GV) or metaphase II (MII) stage of nuclear maturity

2. cryopreservation of immature primordial oocytes *in situ* in fragments of ovarian cortex (Picton, Gosden and Leibo 2003).

Cryopreservation of secondary oocytes

Although it has proved possible to obtain live births after the frozen storage of mouse oocytes, human oocytes generally have a low post-thaw survival and developmental potential. Consequently, only a small number of babies have been born worldwide from thousands of frozen-thawed oocytes and the live birth rate, even in healthy women, is still very low (Porcu *et al.* 2000). These disappointing success rates can be attributed in part to the biological properties of oocytes, as human eggs are extremely sensitive to both temperature and toxic shocks, have a short fertile lifespan and have little capacity for repairing damage. The freeze-thaw process can lead to depolarization of the meiotic spindle microtubules[5] and disruption of chromatid (strands of chromosome) separation at the moment of fertilization with the potential induction of aneuploidy[6] after the extrusion of the second polar body (Miller *et al.* 2004; Mullen *et al.* 2004; Shaw, Oranratnachai and Trounson 2000). Any step in the freeze-thaw process can therefore compromise the meiotic progression and fertile potential of the oocyte (Smith and Silva 2004).

Some of the problems associated with MII oocyte cryopreservation can be overcome by freezing oocytes at the GV stage of nuclear maturity. At this stage of development the chromosomes are decondensed and enclosed in the nuclear envelope and the temperature-sensitive spindle apparatus has not yet formed. Although some encouraging results have been obtained after GV freezing (Goud *et al.* 2000; Tucker *et al.* 1998), this procedure requires the oocytes to undergo nuclear maturation *in vitro* post-thaw, before the oocytes are competent to be fertilized. *In vitro* maturation (IVM) is still regarded by the majority of reproductive medicine practitioners as an experimental technique, which itself is far from optimized (Picton 2002).

Despite the problems associated with GV and MII oocyte freezing, recent modifications in the protocols used for both slow freezing (Borini *et al.* 2004; Fabbri *et al.* 2001) and ultra-rapid freezing or vitrification (Vieira *et al.* 2002; Yoon *et al.* 2003) have led to improved post-thaw survival and fertility of these gametes. Secondary oocyte freezing is therefore becoming a realistic option for those, such as young cancer patients, who have only one chance to freeze their gametes before they start their cancer therapy. While there can be little doubt that the yields of full-sized oocytes for freezing will be highest if the patient undergoes a full programme of ovarian stimulation prior to oocyte harvest, it is possible to use ultrasound-guided trans-vaginal recovery techniques to collect four to six, GV-staged cumulus-enclosed oocytes from unstimulated ovaries on days seven to ten of the reproductive cycle (Wynn *et al.* 1998). Furthermore, the yield of oocytes can be increased marginally to eight to ten with only a short three-day course of FSH stimulation (Wynn *et al.* 1998). Cumulus-enclosed GV oocytes can then be collected and either cryopreserved immediately or matured to MII over 30–36 hours *in vitro* and stored after either slow freezing or vitrification.

The combination of IVM of oocytes and MII oocyte vitrification appears to be a particularly attractive option as a means to preserve the fertility of adolescent patients because this approach can be used to harvest oocytes from follicles of ≥ 4 mm diameter in an unstimulated ovary. This means that oocyte collection can be implemented rapidly without the need for long delays and extended ovarian hyperstimulation. In support of this idea, there are already a small number of ongoing pregnancies in Canada following the vitrification of MII-staged IVM eggs harvested from cancer patients (Tan 2004).

Cryopreservation of primordial oocytes

A radical alternative strategy to secondary oocyte harvesting and banking, which can be used by young girls as well as adolescents and adults irrespective of diagnosis, is the cryopreservation of ovarian tissue (Picton, Kim and Gosden 2000). Compared with the ethical dilemmas of embryo cryopreservation and the technical problems of freezing mature oocytes, ovarian freezing represents an attractive general strategy because it completely removes the germ cells from exposure to harmful cytotoxic agents. Ovarian tissue banking has the added advantage that it offers the patient the potential to restore their natural fertility at a later date through autografting (Donnez *et al.* 2004; Gosden *et al.* 1994; Newton *et al.* 1996) or through the growth of the tissue to maturity *in vitro* (Picton, Harris and Chambers 2004; Figure 5.1). The practice of ovarian tissue cryopreservation is also compatible with the methods proposed above for secondary oocyte harvest and freezing.

Unlike secondary oocyte freezing, the technology of ovarian tissue banking involves freezing immature primordial follicles *in situ* in slices of ovarian cortex (Picton *et al.* 2000; Gosden *et al.* 1994; Newton *et al.* 1996). The harvesting and freeze-storage of ovarian tissue for oncology patients has proved surprisingly easy to do as the outer region of the ovarian cortex contains tens to hundreds or even thousands of primordial and primary follicles, depending on the mass of tissue and age of the patient (Faddy *et al.* 1992). Paradoxically, while primordial follicles are a more effective subject for tissue banking than secondary oocytes, animal studies have demonstrated that it is precisely this stage of follicle development that is most susceptible to the effects of ionizing radiation and alkylating agents (Meirow *et al.* 1999b). Furthermore, a number of studies, including a recent case report of human autografting (see Figure 5.1) after cryopreservation (Radford *et al.* 2001), suggest that the restoration of fertility after ovarian freezing and grafting may be severely compromised by prior exposure to chemo- or radiotherapies before tissue harvesting.

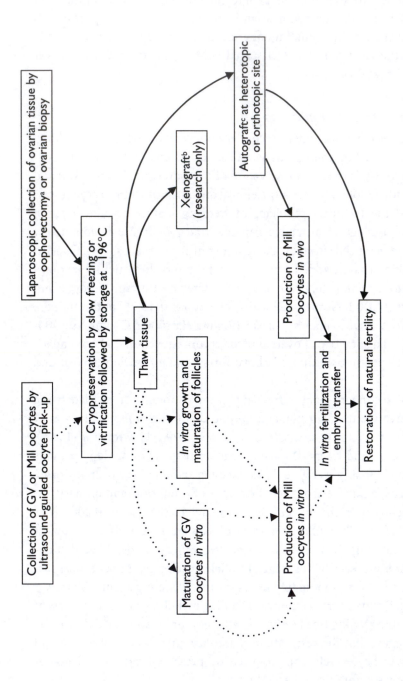

Figure 5.1 Strategies used to cryopreserve and restore female fertility

Notes

a Surgery to remove one or both ovaries.

b Cells of one species transplanted to another species.

c Tissue from one site to another in the same individual.

Ovarian cortex can be harvested relatively quickly, by laparoscopy, laparotomy or oophorectomy (see Figure 5.1), all without the need for any ovarian stimulation (Meirow *et al.* 1999a). The primordial follicles can then be cryopreserved *in situ* within thin (1–2 mm thick) slices of the ovarian cortex using slow freezing techniques without loss of tissue viability (Newton *et al.* 1996) and tissue can be stored indefinitely at liquid nitrogen temperatures.

Restoration of fertility

At present our ability to preserve and store ovarian cortex is far ahead of the development of the methods that are needed to realize the fertile potential of this tissue. Two approaches are being explored at the present time.

Autografting

To date, the most viable clinical option for fertility restoration in girls and young women after ovarian tissue cryopreservation is centred around orthotopic or heterotopic autografting of cryopreserved tissue (Figure 5.1). Indeed there have now been a number of reported cases of a transient restoration of follicle growth in young women after ovarian autografting (for example, Oktay and Yih 2002; Oktay *et al.* 2004; Radford *et al.* 2001). The most recent reported case resulted in the birth of a healthy baby girl to a 26-year-old Belgium woman who had tissue from one of her ovaries cryopreserved prior to chemotherapy for Hodgkin's lymphoma (Donnez *et al.* 2004). The successful development of this technology in humans follows the restoration of natural fertility and the birth of live young in a number of species including sheep (Gosden *et al.* 1994; Salle *et al.* 2003) and rabbits (Almodin *et al.* 2004) after autografting of cryopreserved ovarian tissue. In all of the species studied to date, autografting resulted in only a temporary restoration of ovarian function for, although the majority (90–95%) of the follicles are likely to be viable following freezing and thawing (Newton *et al.* 1996), a far smaller proportion (35–50%) of these follicles is likely to survive the reduced oxygen state associated with revascularization of the grafted tissue (Nugent *et al.* 1998). Many questions must therefore be answered before cryopreservation and autografting can be considered a reliable means of preserving and restoring the fertility of young patients.

Follicle culture

While autografting shows significant promise as a means to restore fertility, where there is any risk of reintroducing malignant cells in the graft to a young patient, such as in the case of blood-borne diseases and ste-roid-related cancers (Kim *et al.* 2001; Shaw and Trounson 1997), it is in both the patient's and clinician's best interests to use an alternative strategy. It may, for example, be possible to purge the ovarian tissue of tumour cell contamination using *in vitro* culture techniques (Schroder *et al.* 2004) before autografting. Alternatively, the complete *in vitro* growth (IVG) and matura-tion of cryopreserved follicles may be the safest way to proceed (Picton *et al.* 2004). In the latter strategy, the follicles contained in the frozen-thawed tis-sue must be grown to maturity *in vitro* before the mature eggs can be fertilized and the embryos, which are free from contamination, can then be transferred back to the patient. If successful and efficient, the complete IVG of human oocytes from cryopreserved ovarian cortex may eventually super-sede autografting as the safest strategy to restore natural fertility. However, to achieve this goal, a considerable amount of research must be conducted to confirm that ovarian cryopreservation followed by extended follicle culture is both an efficient and safe procedure and does not induce genetic and epigenetic[7] alterations in the oocytes and embryos so derived as a direct result of either the freeze-thawing process or as a consequence of extended culture (Reik and Walter 2001; Young and Fairburn 2000). A number of parameters must be considered before an effective IVG strategy can be implemented.

Any culture strategy designed to support the complete IVG of oocytes and follicles from cryopreserved tissues must mimic the sequence of events and cellular checkpoints that the follicles and oocytes would normally be exposed to *in vivo*. The growth rates, cell–cell signalling and metabolic turn-over of follicles and oocytes grown *in vitro* must correspond to the parame-ters of similar cells grown to maturity in the body. During their extended growth phase, oocytes progressively synthesize and accumulate the payload of proteins and acids (RNAs), which are required to support production of a fertile gamete and the pre-implantation development of the early embryo (Picton, Briggs and Gosden 1998). Furthermore, there are stage-specific changes in genomic imprinting during oocyte growth *in vivo* that must be replicated in oocytes grown *in vitro* (Huntriss *et al.* 2004; Mertineit *et al.* 1998).

Despite these stringent biological requirements, significant advances have been made in IVG technologies (see Picton *et al.* 2004 for review). Encouraging results have been obtained in laboratory species (O'Brien, Pendola and Eppig 2003). In contrast, progress in IVG in large animals and humans is far slower than that observed in rodents, as ruminant and human oocytes are much larger eggs, which take many months to acquire their fertile potential (Newton, Picton and Gosden 1999; Picton *et al.* 2004). Nevertheless, in both sheep and humans it is now possible to: initiate and maintain primordial follicle growth over extended periods; induce antral cavity formation in preantral follicles; induce appropriate levels of steroid biosynthesis after provision of suitable substrates (Hovatta *et al.* 1999; Newton *et al.* 1999; Picton *et al.* 2003). Importantly, extensive validation studies carried out on isolated sheep follicles have revealed that IVG can be achieved with equal efficiency using both fresh and cryopreserved tissue. Electron microscopy has also shown that the *in vitro*-grown cells have a similar morphology to oocytes and follicles grown *in vivo* (Jin, Harris and Picton 2004). Further advances in IVG technology will soon enable us to determine if the oocytes derived following cryopreservation and IVG of human ovarian cortex are healthy and fertile.

Future prospects

Loss of ovarian function and reduction of fertile potential in young patients can be combated by the development of strategies to quantify the risk of ovarian damage, to protect the gonads from the destructive effects of medical treatments and, in extreme cases, to cryopreserve fertility. Advances in fertility preservation methods for young patients will inevitably be dependent on the development of an improved understanding of the effects on the ovary of contemporary treatments, as exposure to cytotoxic agents is frequently unavoidable prior to a window of safety being available for oocyte and ovarian tissue harvesting. Furthermore, the development of a safe clinical strategy to preserve the fertility of all young patients, irrespective of diagnosis, has to be based around high-quality basic research into the biology and technology of oocyte and ovarian tissue cryopreservation and its safe and efficient use to restore fertility. Future research topics are therefore likely to include: development of new diagnostics to test the gonadotoxicity of treatments such as those offered to cancer patients; development of accurate methods to predict the lifespan of autografts; determination of the optimum location of autografts; assessment of the impact of patient age on

the efficiency of the freezing, thawing and grafting or IVG processes; quanti-
fication of the consequences of prior exposure to chemo- or radiotherapies;
and evaluation of the normality of uterine function and the contribution of
the uterus to implantation post-treatment.

Notes

1 Family of anticancer drugs that interferes with the cell's DNA and inhibits
  cancer cell growth.
2 Absent or decreased function of the male testis or female ovary (gonads).
3 Compound important in the metabolism of nerve cells.
4 Destructive of bone marrow activity.
5 Protein scaffold on which the chromosomes are aligned during the process of
  cell division which produces a fertile egg.
6 Variation in chromosome number involving one or a small number of
  chromosomes. Commonly involves the gain or loss of a single chromosome.
7 Something that affects a cell without affecting its DNA.

6.

Fertility Preservation Methods and Treatments for Males

Allan Pacey

Introduction

Techniques for the fertility preservation in males are almost exclusively based around the ability to freeze spermatozoa and cryopreserve them in liquid nitrogen until such time that they can be used in an assisted conception procedure. Although the ability to freeze human sperm was first demonstrated in the late eighteenth century, its application to fertility preservation prior to potentially sterilizing medical treatments did not occur until the mid-nineteenth century. Since that time, there have been many advances both in the technology used to freeze and store sperm, as well as that which allows it to be used to achieve a pregnancy. This chapter will review the current state of the art of fertility preservation in males by sperm freezing as well as look to the future for possible developments in this area.

The process of sperm banking

The ability to freeze sperm and place it in storage relies on being able to obtain a suitable sample of spermatozoa from the patient. In the first instance, this almost always requires the patient to be able to provide a semen sample by masturbation. Unfortunately, there are some patients for whom masturbation to orgasm is simply not possible, either because they are feeling too ill to become sexually aroused or because physiological changes due to their disease – or the side-effects of treatment or surgery – prevent them being able to achieve an erection or ejaculate (see Tomlinson and Pacey 2003). In these cases, alternative strategies to obtain sperm can be considered (Table 6.1), although often the time pressures to begin treatment (in the case of cancer treatments for example), and the additional risks that these procedures sometimes carry to the patient's health, can preclude them from being used routinely.

Assuming the patient is able to masturbate a sample for cryopreservation and that he has gone through puberty, then the medical evidence to date would suggest that, at least in cancer patients, the semen quality is broadly similar across disease states (Bahadur *et al.* 2002) and is comparable to that of males without malignancies (Rofeim and Gilbert 2004). However, there will inevitably be some patients where no (or too few) sperm can be obtained for freezing, either from an initial masturbatory ejaculate or from a more sophisticated (sperm retrieval) technique (see Table 6.1). Azoospermia[1] may occur for a variety of reasons relating to an inherent underlying genetic condition that is independent of the disease state under treatment, or due to a direct physiological association with it.

**Table 6.1 Techniques of non-surgical
and surgical methods of sperm recovery**

Non-surgical methods	
Method	*Description*
Recovery of sperm from post-masturbatory urine	In men with retrograde ejaculation at orgasm, sperm enter the bladder rather than out of the penis but viable sperm can be recovered from alkalinized urine for cryopreservation
Sildenafil Citrate (Viagra)	Useful for patients who encounter temporary erectile dysfunction at the time of sample production. The effect is short-lived and has been shown to be of some value in IVF cycles
Electrovibration stimulation	Electrovibration stimulation of the penis initiates reflex spinal cord activity causing ejaculation
Trans-rectal electroejaculation	This stimulates the nerves responsible for ejaculation but it is not without risk of injury to the rectal mucosa or, more seriously, autonomic dysreflexia,[a] which is potentially life threatening

Continued on next page

Table 6.1 cont.

Surgical methods

Site of recovery	Description
Vas deferens Vas deferens sperm extraction	Rarely performed but can be used as an alternative to electroejaculation. Now largely replaced by sperm extraction from the epididymis or testicles
Epididymis Micro-epididymal sperm aspiration (MESA)	Involves surgical exploration, and exposure of the testes and epididymis from the scrotum. Usually performed in an operating theatre under general anaesthetic
Percutaneous[b] epididymal sperm aspiration (PESA)	Sperm are removed from the epididymis by a needle inserted through the scrotum. Less invasive than MESA with fewer complications and usually performed as a day case
Testicles Testicular sperm aspiration (TESA)	Sperm extraction is performed percutaneously under local anaesthetic using a needle
Testicular sperm extraction (TESE)	A piece of testicular tissue is recovered as a biopsy and sperm recovered by micro-dissection in the laboratory. Requires exposure of an area of the testis, but post-operative complications are rare

Notes

a Potentially dangerous complications of a spinal cord injury, often involving dangerously high blood pressure.

b Through the skin.

Freezing and long-term storage of sperm

The science that underpins successful sperm cryopreservation has been reviewed many times (see Fuller and Paynter 2004) and involves a complex understanding of physics and biology. However, in simple terms, cryo-storage is able to keep sperm in a state of 'suspended animation'. The ability to keep sperm frozen in this state relies upon the addition of a cryo-protectant to the sperm sample before it is cooled to the required temperature. While there are a number of different formulations of cryo-protectant on the market, they all act in a very similar way and essentially work to dehydrate the spermatozoa and in doing so protect it from the formation of intracellular ice, which can be lethal to living cells upon thawing. Crucial to the process is the requirement to lower the temperature of the sperm/cryoprotectant mixture very slowly and in a controlled way. While the majority of clinics still freeze sperm by crudely suspending the samples to be frozen in nitrogen vapour (Sherman 1963), better success rates (in terms of post-thaw survival – see below) have been obtained using controlled rate freezers (Ragni *et al.* 1990) where the temperature gradient can be controlled more precisely.

Although the precise details of the technical system used to freeze and store spermatozoa will be variable from laboratory to laboratory according to personal preferences and historical factors, it will almost certainly involve the decision to hold the sperm/cryoprotectant mixture in a series of plastic straws or ampoules (Figures 6.1 and 6.2) and to maintain the temperature of the frozen material in either the liquid or vapour phase of liquid nitrogen (see Mortimer 1994 for review). The exact number of vials or straws obtained from a single ejaculate is variable and is dependent on a number of factors including the volume of the ejaculate produced, the type of freezing protocol used (which determines the volume of cryoprotectant added) and the type of vial or straw selected. However, as a general rule, assuming there is sufficient volume before freezing, each ejaculate would normally be divided into smaller aliquots to provide a number of attempts at conception (depending on the technique required – see below).

When a decision has been taken to freeze spermatozoa in straws, then these are normally stored submerged in liquid nitrogen (at -196°C) whereas those keeping samples in liquid nitrogen vapour (at -140°C or below) will generally use ampoules. In either case, the important point is that the spermatozoa are kept at a constant temperature of below the recrystallization point of pure water at -130°C. It is for this reason that storage vessels (liquid or vapour) need to be checked regularly and are usually fitted with alarm systems to warn staff if the temperature rises above predetermined levels. Vapour phase systems often have electronic auto-fill mechanisms whereby the vessel is automatically topped up with more nitrogen as required, whereas liquid phase vessels (often called dewars) usually need to be topped up manually every few days (although they can stand for many weeks and maintain their temperature).

A common question about freezing sperm is, how long can sperm be held in the frozen state yet still be thawed and then used to achieve a viable

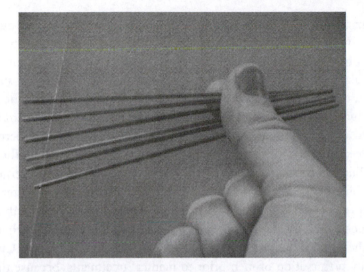

Figure 6.1 Photograph of six 0.5 ml straws that are commonly used to freeze aliquots of human semen during sperm banking. After filling, the open end of the straw is filled with a 'sealing powder' that polymerizes at low temperature thereby keeping the frozen contents inside the straw during long-term storage in liquid nitrogen

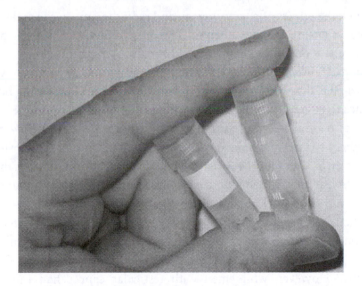

Figure 6.2 Photographs of two plastic ampoules used to freeze and store aliquots of human semen during sperm banking. After filling, the ampoule is sealed with a screw top. Two different sizes of ampoules are shown holding 1.0 ml (left) and 2.0 ml (right) of semen respectively

pregnancy and healthy birth? At the time of writing, the longest duration between sperm banking and conception is 21 years as evidenced by a case report of a young man who stored sperm at age 17 prior to treatment for testicular cancer and then, after being found to be azoospermic,[1] successfully used the samples to achieve a conception with his partner at the age of 38 (Horne *et al.* 2004). It is only a matter of time before this record is surpassed and from a theoretical standpoint there is no reason why sperm may not be kept frozen for much longer and still remain functional. In the cattle breeding industry, for example, it is known anecdotally that sperm from some bulls has been successfully used to sire calves over 40 years after it was first frozen! However, such data remains unpublished and there are theoretical concerns as to the integrity of the nuclear DNA in samples that have been held in storage for a long period of time. This is particularly relevant to fertility preservation of men prior to medical treatments, because there is some evidence to suggest that the process of freezing and thawing itself can lead to DNA damage in sperm, at least in infertile men (Donnelly *et al.* 2001).

Conception following medical treatments

Although the effects of chemotherapy and radiotherapy on the male reproductive system are well documented (Howell and Shalet 1998), the precise effects on any one individual remain difficult to predict.

For males who are already producing sperm at the time of diagnosis and treatment (i.e. they have passed through puberty) there is a growing body of evidence to suggest that, for some treatments at least, there can be a good chance of natural fertility returning in the months or years following the cessation of treatment. For example, in an examination of 1115 post-treatment semen analyses in 314 patients who had received gonadotoxic therapy over a 26-year period, Bahadur *et al.* (2005) found that the type of cancer (or disease) and the initial pre-treatment sperm concentration were the most significant factors governing post-treatment semen quality and the recovery of spermatogenesis. For example, patients with lymphoma and leukaemia had the highest incidence of post-treatment azoospermia and oligozoospermia.[2] However, while men with testicular cancer had the lowest pre-treatment sperm concentrations, they also had the lowest incidence of azoospermia after treatment. This confirms an earlier observation by Lampe *et al.* (1997) who in a follow-up study of 178 men after chemotherapy treatment for testicular germ cell cancer found that 80 per cent of men had recovered some sperm production after five years since chemotherapy with 60 per cent reaching normal levels. Across all disease states Bahadur *et al.* (2005) concluded that only 37 per cent of patients had permanent post-treatment azoospermia, which goes some way to explain why relatively few males return to use their sperm-banked samples in future years (see below) – that is, because the majority are able to conceive quite naturally with no need for medical assistance.

For males who were treated at an earlier age, however (i.e. before the onset of puberty), the received wisdom is often that the pre-pubertal testis is less susceptible to damage by gonadotoxic agents and therefore the boy's fertility is less likely to be affected when he reaches adulthood. However, the evidence to support this point of view is lacking and it has been suggested that there may still be sufficient cellular activity in the apparently quiescent (pre-pubertal) testis (Chemes 2001) for significant gonadotoxic damage to occur (Wallace, Anderson and Irvine 2005). This is exemplified by a number of studies that have looked at the adult semen quality of childhood cancer survivors. For example, Lopez Andreu *et al.* (2000) and Relander *et al.* (2000) followed two independent cohorts (various diagnoses) of boys for over 13+ years and found that only 37 per cent and 63 per cent respectively had normal spermatogenesis as adults. Similarly, a study of 33 males with a history of childhood cancer (with a median age at diagnosis of ten years old) found that only 33 per cent had normal semen quality as adults and 30 per cent were azoospermic (Thomson *et al.* 2002). By contrast, a study by Byrne *et al.* (2004) of survivors of childhood acute lymphoblastic leukaemia found that only men treated with high-dose cranial radiotherapy had a significantly reduced fertility when compared with controls. Ironically, in those who were treated as pre-pubertal boys and who have permanent azoospermia as adults, there are very few options to assist with their infertility because they will not have had the opportunity to bank sperm prior to the onset of treatment. This represents significant challenges for the medical and scientific community as the survival rates of childhood cancer continue to improve (Wallace *et al.* 2005).

For adult males who are intending to conceive with their partner, irrespective of whether they had medical treatments before or after puberty, the general opinion is that if normal levels of sperm production are occurring at the time that conception is being considered, then there should be no reason why the couple should not be able to conceive by methods of natural family planning and with no medical intervention. This is notwithstanding that the probability of sub-fertility in the female partner will be evident at a level consistent with the general population of pregnancy planners and this in itself may require the couple to need some form of assisted conception to overcome it (see below). Unfortunately, the actual incidence of unassisted conception in men with a previous cancer diagnosis has not been systematically described for all medical conditions and treatment options. However, over a ten-year follow-up period of men with stage 1 testis tumour Herr *et al.* (1998) indicated that 65 per cent of couples that attempted a pregnancy were successful. In a further series of 63 patients with testicular germ cell malignancy (Jacobsen *et al.* 2002) 40 per cent of patients who attempted fatherhood were successful at initiating a pregnancy (although only 24% were without the assistance of assisted conception).

Methods of assisted conception

Should methods of natural family planning fail then there are currently a number of methods of assisted conception that can be used. These are summarized in Table 6.2 and range from a relatively simple and inexpensive procedure such as intra-uterine insemination (IUI) to more sophisticated procedures such as *in vitro* fertilization (IVF) and intra-cytoplasmic sperm injection (ICSI). The choice of which technique to use (for any couple) is dependent on a range of factors and includes the:

1. quality (and quantity) of the sperm available (freshly ejaculated or cryopreserved)

2. physiology of the female partner

3. choice of the patients

4. funding available to the patient.

With regard to the latter point, it is a sad reflection that in circumstances where public money is unavailable to fund treatment and the couple needs to fund their own, then the choice of treatment may be sometimes dictated by the cost rather than its clinical effectiveness. However, little has been published on this topic and so it remains anecdotal as to whether the availability of funding is a major factor in influencing the outcome of fertility treatment in this group of patients.

In the context of this chapter, the treatments shown in Table 6.2 are broadly listed in the order of their clinical effectiveness in dealing with sperm-related problems (i.e. the quality of the semen samples available for

Table 6.2 Techniques of assisted conception applicable for men with semen samples frozen prior to medical treatments

Method	Details	Approximate number of motile sperm required
Intra-cervical insemination (IC)	Involves the insemination into the cervical canal of the female partner of semen that has been thawed. This is rarely performed with ovarian stimulation in the partner. Has been largely replaced by IUI	> 5,000,000
Intra-uterine insemination (IUI)	Thawed spermatozoa are prepared by centrifugation to remove them from seminal plasma. They are re-suspended in a volume of tissue culture fluid and introduced into the uterine cavity of the female partner. Usually done in combination with ovarian stimulation	> 5,000,000
Gametes intra fallopian transfer (GIFT)	Thawed sperm are prepared as in IUI and eggs are recovered from the female partner (as in IVF) and both are introduced into the Fallopian tube during a surgical procedure. Now rarely performed but useful in patients who have ethical objections to IVF and the creation of embryos *in vitro*	> 10,000
Zygote intra fallopian transfer (ZIFT)	Eggs are fertilized *in vitro* with prepared (thawed) sperm (as in IVF) but the fertilized egg is returned to the Fallopian tube where subsequent development can take place. Has the advantage over GIFT in that fertilization can be confirmed, but a disadvantage in comparison to IVF since embryo development is not observed. Now rarely performed	> 10,000
In vitro fertilization (IVF)	Eggs are recovered from the female partner following ovarian stimulation. Prepared frozen sperm are used to fertilize them *in vitro*. Resulting embryos are cultured for between two and five days with the best two or three replaced in the uterine cavity. Supernumerary embryos can be frozen and potentially replaced later	> 10,000
Intra-cytoplasmic sperm injection (ICSI)	Procedurally almost identical to IVF, except that a single spermatozoon is injected directly into the egg cytoplasm. Ideally motile sperm are selected but in very poor samples immotile but viable (living) sperm can be injected. Requires only enough viable sperm as there are eggs available for injection	10–10,000

treatment). As such, there are very different treatment options available for a man who has some recovery of spermatogenesis following a medical treatment compared with a man who might be azoospermic after treatment and only have the limited resource of his frozen samples in storage.

For example, for a man who, at the time of entering an assisted conception programme with his partner, is ejaculating moderate number of motile spermatozoa and from whose ejaculates at least five million motile sperm per millilitre can be prepared, a relatively simple procedure such as IUI using freshly ejaculated sperm would seem most appropriate. Whereas in a man whose ejaculates have been consistently azoospermic but who has frozen samples from which at least 10 or 20 motile sperm can be identified, then ICSI would certainly be required. However, in reality this is a somewhat simple way of looking at the decision as in each case account needs to be taken of the biology of the man's partner and there are many circumstances where the aggressiveness of the assisted conception treatment has to be increased because of pathological factors on the female side. For example, previous disease or damage to the Fallopian tubes will almost certainly require the couple to use IVF even if the quality of sperm available would be sufficient for IUI in another woman.

An interesting question is the decision that is made surrounding the use of fresh or frozen sperm in cases where the quality of the two (in terms of the concentration of motile sperm) is very similar post-treatment. Anecdotally, opinion is divided as to which is the better option, the anxiety being that following any medical treatments involving cytotoxic drugs there is a known increase in sperm chromosomal abnormalities that theoretically could lead to an increase in spontaneous abortions, stillbirths or birth defects in children (Hassold *et al.* 1996). However, although an increase in sperm chromosomal abnormalities has been observed in men during and immediately following treatment (Robbins *et al.* 1997), it is generally considered that this is transient and that as soon as six months after the treatment has ended (Meistrich 1993) it is safe for a couple to attempt pregnancy, either naturally or with assisted conception techniques. Although more recent data has suggested that sperm aneuploidy (having one or more extra or missing chromosomes leading to an unbalanced chromosome complement) may persist until at least 18 months post-treatment (De Mas *et al.* 2001), there is no evidence from long-term follow-up studies (Byrne *et al.* 1998) that the offspring of those treated with potentially mutagenic therapies have a significant increase in genetic disease.

Finally, in those men who were permanently azoospermic following medical treatment with gonadotoxic agents and where there was no (or very poor quality) sperm stored, there has historically been no effective treatment options available to them apart from considering the use of donor sperm. However, the recent advances combining testicular sperm extraction (see Table 6.1) with ICSI (Table 6.2) has led to some interesting and useful options for these men. At the time of writing there are at least four studies (Chan *et al.* 2001; Damani *et al.* 2002; Meseguer *et al.* 2003; Tournaye 2000) in which sperm could be recovered in between 40 per cent and 65 per cent of patients using techniques of testicular biopsy. In some instances the use of these sperm in ICSI has led to live births. Clearly, in these instances the same concerns of the possibility of sperm chromosomal damage are relevant and would need to be considered before these sperm are used in treatment.

Future developments in fertility preservation in males

Although the cryopreservation of ejaculated (or surgically recovered) mature spermatozoa remains the mainstay of fertility preservation in males, there are a number of areas of current research which, if successful, could revolutionize fertility preservation.

The first is based on an approach to try and actually prevent the death or damage to the population of stem (sperm-producing) cells in the testis that typically occurs following exposure to radiation or alkylating agents (see above). Following a number of experimental observations in rats, it has been suggested that this might be possible by altering the endocrine environment (essentially suppressing the production of testosterone and follicle stimulating hormone or FSH) of the patient either before or after the onset of treatment (Meistrich and Shetty 2003). However, although this strategy can restore some sperm production in the rat, it is not yet known whether it can be adapted for human clinical application. Encouraging results from a small study of 15 patients with nephritic syndrome[3] (being treated with the chemotherapy drug cyclophosphamide) have been obtained (Masala *et al.* 1997). More recent experiments in non-human primates (Boekelheide *et al.* 2005) have, however, been unable to reproduce the experimental results obtained in rats, raising the possibility that there are important species-specific differences in the testicular response either to the treatment (in this case radiotherapy) or the endocrine rescue protocol, or both. As an approach, therefore, the use of endocrine manipulation to protect the testis from damage (or salvage them from it) is still very much experimental.

A second area of research activity is in the area of spermatogonial transplantation. Unlike the current approach of freezing mature ejaculated sperm, many authors have commented on the desirability of being able to remove (before treatment) and potentially replace (after treatment) a population of the stem (sperm-producing) cells (called spermatogonia) within the testis that ultimately give rise to sperm. The advantage of being able to do this is that, unlike frozen sperm that are a finite resource, stem cells in the testis are 'self-renewing'. As such, if they could be successfully transplanted back into the patient, then they could continue to produce sperm for the rest of his life. Even if this was only moderately successful, then it could potentially provide sufficient (freshly ejaculated) sperm for use in repeated cycles of assisted conception. If very successful, and ejaculates were near normal in terms of quality, then it is possible to envisage some patients being able to father a child quite normally and without further assistance.

Although the concept of spermatogonial transplantation remained theoretical for many years, major progress was made when Brinster and Zimmermann (1994) published details of experiments in mice where they had successfully removed spermatogonia from one individual and transplanted it back into the testes of another animal. This provided proof of concept that the technique was feasible, and, in subsequent years, the underlying technology for retrieval, storage, genetic manipulation (important for animal breeding purposes) and transplantation were developed (see Johnson, Russell and Griswold 2000). In progressing to human clinical trials scientists have been notably cautious. Although some small-scale trials have been attempted (Radford, Shalet and Lieberman 1999), at the time of writing the results have not yet been published.

A major concern with this approach, however, is the fear that in oncology patients in particular, the process of transplantation could lead to the re-introduction of malignant cells into the patient who was otherwise cured of his original disease. It has been suggested that this is particularly pertinent for lymphoma and leukaemia patients as in these diseases the testis is a likely organ for the settlement of metastasizing cells (Schlatt 2002) as has been shown experimentally in leukaemic rats (Jahnukainen *et al.* 2001). This could be potentially avoided if it were possible to develop suitable technologies by which the process of spermatogenesis could occur *in vitro*.

The prospects for spermatogenesis *in vitro* have recently been reviewed by Parks *et al.* (2003) who outline the technical complexity of cell culture systems that would be required to maintain the development of spermatozoa *in vitro*. Although some progress in animal models has been made (in as much as presumptive spermatids [i.e. early sperm cells] expressing appropriate genetic markers have been identified and have been injected into eggs to produce viable embryos), it is far from the stage of being clinically useful for human applications. However, an area with perhaps more technical promise is in the development of techniques to transplant pieces of testicular material (termed explants) into 'host' animals that then act to support the sperm production process. Proof that this can work has come from a number of experimental approaches (reviewed in Parks *et al.* 2003) dating back to the 1970s and interestingly it seems as though spermatogenesis can be supported even when testicular explants are transplanted to various extra-testicular sites. More recently Honaramooz *et al.* (2002) were able to show that this technique could be used to initiate spermatogenesis in pre-pubertal testicular tissue, which could give hope for fertility preservation in pre-pubertal boys where sperm banking is not possible (see above). However, it should be recognized that this type of xenotransplantation may raise many ethical issues in some individuals, and there are obvious safety concerns to address about the potential for non-human DNA (or animal viruses) being transferred to the fertilized egg during the assisted conception procedure. Much work is therefore needed until the safety and acceptability of this approach can be demonstrated.

Concluding remarks

Fertility preservation in males has a long history and sperm banks were in existence well before the development of the sophisticated assisted conception technologies (e.g. IVF and ICSI) that are now used to provide the opportunity for men rendered infertile through medical treatments to father their own genetic child. However, it should be recognized that the process of sperm banking is much more than just the provision of infertility treatment to males who have stored sperm prior to medical treatments. It involves an ongoing interaction with the patient in the years post-banking to review his fertility after treatment has ceased and provide practical and ongoing advice about contraception, family planning, access to counselling and assisted conception treatments, if that is required. Sadly, this is sometimes forgotten by staff in many IVF units who provide sperm banking services alongside their repertoire of infertility treatments yet provide little by the way of a focused service for men in the years between banking and assisted conception treatment (Tomlinson and Pacey 2003).

For men banking sperm, there may be complex reasons why they are placing their sperm in storage that are unrelated to the process of becoming a father (Pacey 2003). As such, their immediate needs may well be more for support and advice regarding their reproductive function and fertility (including contraception) rather than about assisted conception procedures. Indeed, the evidence shows that of the many men who store sperm, only a small proportion (10 to 25%) ever request to attempt to achieve a pregnancy with their frozen samples (Blackhall *et al.* 2002; Kelleher *et al.* 2001). While some may view this as disappointing, it may well reflect the fact that in many men, spermatogenesis remains unaffected or is only temporarily suppressed and recovers sufficiently to allow them to achieve conception with their partner without the need for medical assistance. In spite of the obvious success of modern assisted conception techniques, this is surely the method by which most men and their partners would prefer to conceive.

Notes

1 Where no sperm is present in the ejaculate.
2 Having less than 20 million sperm per millimetre of semen.
3 Inflammation of the kidneys that damages the filtering mechanisms.

7.

Legal and Ethical Aspects Surrounding Fertility Preservation Services for Children and Young People

David Green and Marilyn Crawshaw

Introduction

There are still only a few jurisdictions in the world that regulate assisted conception and fertility preservation services. Debates about the need for regulation reflect some of the tensions that exist within this controversial area of medicine. Professional self-regulation systems exist in a number of countries, supported by those who argue that only experts in the field can understand the complexity of the issues and practices and/or those who contend that the involvement of the state would amount to social engineering. Even in countries such as the UK, which offer state-provided health care and state-sanctioned regulation, private health care is typically a major provider of assisted conception services and there are often differences in the regulation systems of the two sectors. Private health care is arguably more heavily influenced by commercial and financial considerations, whereas state health care is more susceptible to the political climate. In countries where there is a dominant religious presence, this too can influence the relevant legislative framework. Finally, differences in cultural approaches to science can contribute to the global patchwork quilt effect of both service provision and regulation.

As the UK was the first country to bring in legal regulation of assisted conception services and remains the flagship, this chapter will concentrate on the UK regulatory scene as a backdrop to considering some of the ethical issues arising from the provision of fertility preservation services to those who have not yet attained the age of majority.

Legal framework

The Human Fertilisation and Embryology Act entered the UK statute books in 1990 and was implemented on 1 August 1991. It covers the majority of, though not all, assisted conception treatments and requires that centres providing such treatments or carrying out proscribed research should be licensed and inspected annually. It set up a regulatory body – the Human Fertilisation & Embryology Authority (HFEA) – with the function of inspecting centres and issuing licences, producing a Code of Practice, monitoring new developments, consulting with professionals, patients and the general public about whether to license new treatments, publishing patient information and maintaining a Register of Information about treatments and live births.

When the Act was passed, some fertility preservation services were already storing the mature gametes of some patients, including minors, about to enter treatments that might render them infertile (the Act only covers mature gametes: regulation of storage of immature gametes is covered below). However, numbers were low and the Act did not make any special provision for the younger age group.

People facing potentially sterilizing treatments are treated in UK law in the same way as others using fertility preservation services – including couples storing their embryos for future treatment and gamete donors. They are required to have the medical, scientific, legal and psycho-social implications of their decision explained to them, to be offered counselling and to have sufficient time to consider their decision prior to signing an HFEA consent form (HFEA 2003 Part 6). However, there are two notable differences for this group. First, their gametes can be stored up to them reaching age 55 rather than for the usual ten year maximum storage period (or five years for embryos). Second, they have the option to consent either for storage only or for storage and use. If they opt for the former, then the fuller second consent form is completed at a later stage. In practice, their choice may be limited as many assisted conception centres operate their own policy about which form to use. The forms require patients to state their wishes for the disposal of their sperm (including whether or not they agree to it being used for research) in the event of their death or any incapacity that might render them incapable of varying or revoking consent. If the dual purpose form is used, the name of a partner (if any) to whom they give the right to access their sperm and their wishes as to whether they want their name to appear on the register of births and on the birth certificate (Human Fertilisation and Embryology (Deceased Fathers) Act 2003)[1] for any child born following posthumous use of their sperm must be included. Consents may be varied at any time.

The situation is similar for females. However, because storage and treatment using frozen eggs is at a more experimental stage, only a very limited number of centres have been given a storage licence. The more complicated and time-consuming medical procedure required in order to retrieve eggs also means that these services are much less widely used than are sperm storage services (see Chapters 5 and 6).

Many jurisdictions distinguish between minors and those who have attained the age of majority in relation to health care decision-making in general. For example, in England and Wales, those aged 16 and over are presumed to be able to consent to all medical interventions on their own behalf (Family Law Reform Act 1969 s8(1)), providing that they are assessed as being *Gillick* competent (*Gillick* v. *West Norfolk and Wisbech Area Health Authority* 1985 – see below). If they are under 16, it is recommended practice that they are allowed to consent on their own behalf if they are *Gillick* competent but that those with parental responsibility for them should ideally be involved in the decision-making process. Parents can consent on their child's behalf if their child wishes this. In almost all aspects of health care, a parent can legally override their under-age child's decision to refuse treatment (although this is rare) but they cannot override a decision to receive treatment made by their (competent) child (Department of Health 2004a). It is true to say that both The Children Act 1989 and the UN Convention on the Rights of the Child 1989 strengthen the rights of competent young people to have their decisions given due weight (Freeman 1993). However, the unusual legal situation posed by the consent provisions of the HFE Act is that there are *no* circumstances at all in which parents can consent on their child's behalf or override their child's wishes.

Assessment of *Gillick* competence is not without controversy. It was introduced in 1985 as a result of a court case in which a mother disputed the right of her under-age daughter to seek contraceptive advice without her knowledge. The assessment has to be carried out by a medical practitioner (usually the one treating the minor) who has to be satisfied that they have the intellectual capacity to make and express a decision by listening to, and understanding sufficiently, the offered information about the intervention and its consequences and any discussion about it – and to do so voluntarily; that is, without undue influence from family members, professionals or others. Additionally, the HFE Act requirements set out above, including the offer of independent counselling, apply. Clearly, the complexity of the decision to be made may affect the outcome of the assessment, although that is not laid down (Hedley 2000; Wallace and Walker 2001).

This potential for subjective interpretation means that some minors may be excluded from access to storage services if their medical practitioner assesses them as not yet *Gillick* competent, even if another may take a more relaxed stance. There is no available research to indicate whether this is actually happening, though variations in interpretation may go some way to explain the rather patchy provision of services existing both in the UK and North America (Glaser, Wilkey and Greenberg 2000; Glaser *et al.* 2004). There are indications of general professional unease in this area of work and the lack of written guidelines appears to contribute to this (Crawshaw *et al.* 2004; Multi-disciplinary Working Group 2003; Wilford and Hunt 2003).

Minors not yet deemed *Gillick* competent and those who are temporarily mentally incapacitated *but who have mature gametes* may thus be excluded from using storage services. The apparent legal inconsistency between this and other under-age consents is illustrated by the fact that, if surgery or electroejaculation were to be offered as a retrieval method rather than masturbation, then those with parental responsibility for the minor could consent to the anaesthesia and surgery but not to the storage of their son's gametes.

The HFE Act also established another unusual situation with regard to disclosure of information to other parties. Unlike most medical interventions, licensed assisted conception centres cannot disclose information about a patient to anyone not named on their licence without their written consent (HFE Act Section 33). This includes not only the referring doctor and the family doctor but also the parents, even where the child is under 16.

Because of storage infection control requirements, it has been considered good practice for some time to run viral screening tests prior to gametes being stored. This became compulsory from the end of 2004 (HFEA 2001) and throws up particular considerations for those seeking extended storage.

Alongside the pressure of making a decision about storage and acting on it hard on the heels of receiving a diagnosis of serious illness, all patients are now required to give informed consent to screening for hepatitis, HIV and sexually transmitted diseases – a tall order for anyone but perhaps additionally so for those who may be as young as 12 or 13.

Recent years have seen a rapid increase in the storage of the reproductive tissues of younger children. The rather different consent provisions for such storage make for a somewhat anomalous situation when compared with storage of mature gametes.

Consent at any age to the removal of testicular or ovarian tissue for storage is covered by the Human Tissue Act 1961. This means that the usual consent provisions for minors apply rather than the more stringent ones of the HFE Act (providing that the tissue does not contain any mature gametes, in which case the HFE Act applies). Parents holding legal parental responsibility can make 'best interests' consent decisions for their under-age offspring on the grounds that such a decision would ensure improvement or prevention of deterioration in their child's physical or mental health. At a future stage, the responsibility for ongoing storage decisions and any treatment decisions would of course have to pass from parent to child. The HFE Act provisions ensure that parents may not make use of the tissue in fertility treatment against the wishes of their child or in the event of their child's death. Some centres have expressly included this in their in-house consent form to make the situation clear to all concerned (Bahadur, Chatterjee and Ralph 2000).

Since 1 April 2003, reproductive tissue must be stored in tissue banks accredited by the Medicines Control Agency (now the Medicines and Healthcare Products Regulatory Agency – MHRA) under the Department of Health Code of Practice for Tissue Banks (2001). Given the stringency of the accreditation requirements, and taking into account the forthcoming requirements of the European Union Tissues and Cells Directive due to be implemented in April 2006 (though with an extra year's grace for those centres already licensed under national regimes to achieve full compliance), few centres currently offer such a facility. Indeed, there are concerns that some existing storage facilities may not be able to meet the new standards.

After considerable speculation and debate, it was announced in July 2004 that a new UK body is to be formed from a merger of the HFEA and the newly created Human Tissue Authority (which has responsibility for tissue storage) (Department of Health 2004c). This development, together with the pending review of the HFE Act, may lead to some changes in both the legal situation and the regulation provisions, which will, it is hoped, address some of the apparently contradictory legal situations. The ethical and emotional challenges remain.

The complexities of decision-making

When young people themselves, or the parents in the case of a younger child, are faced with the prospect of agreeing to a medical intervention that might preserve their reproductive options in the future, they must contend with many uncertainties. What is the status of the intervention on offer? What are the potential risks and benefits of participating – or not? Who is to make this momentous decision and how might they be best advised?

In addition, there is the potential in fertility preservation services for the blurring of the boundaries between research and treatment. Are young people and parents being asked to opt for an established treatment? Are they being invited to participate in a formal research project?

Research or treatment?

There is a sound scientific basis for the belief that cryopreserved tissue taken from young people prior to treatment for childhood cancer might allow them to beget their own children in the foreseeable future. However, there are many more links to be demonstrated in the evidence chain before these procedures can achieve the status of an established treatment. So the honest way to describe the interventions on offer might be promising, but experimental (Grundy *et al.* 2001a). This is precisely the sort of option offered to individuals who are invited to participate in clinical research trials. Indeed, it is arguable that the improvement in survival rates in childhood cancer over the last three decades is a stunning example of the benefits to be gained by the collaboration of medical scientists and informed patients in formal research trials (Eiser 1998).

Whenever treatment trials are conducted, the researchers are obliged to subject their proposals to external ethical scrutiny. A major concern of any ethics committee will be the manner in which information is to be provided for any potential participants in the study. For example, information sheets will need to be designed to meet the needs of specific groups such as children or those for whom English is not their first language. Usually, steps will be taken to separate therapeutic and research roles so that patients can be confident that decisions about participating in research trials will not jeopardize the quality of their ongoing treatment. Emphasis will be given to the right of any participant (of whatever age) to rescind a decision to become involved in a research project. Overall, great care will have to be taken to ensure that patients appreciate the difference between 'treatment as usual' and informed participation in a formally designed research trial (Grundy *et al.* 2001b).

In each of these scenarios, the family or the individual has difficult choices to make but at least they know where they stand. Consider a third alternative. A clinical team is aware of the promise that cryopreservation procedures might have in safeguarding future procreative options for their young patients. They feel they have a moral responsibility to explain the current position and future possibilities to the families or individuals in their care. However, since they are not working within an agreed research protocol, they have no standardized way of managing the decision-making procedure. Practice inevitably varies as clinicians follow their established consultative styles. A situation already riven with uncertainty becomes even more confused for all concerned.

Risk/benefit analysis

The prize that beckons at the end of the trail that starts with diagnosis is not hard to describe. The medical treatment programme on which the young person is due to embark may ensure their survival at the cost of several significant side-effects. One price that the individual may have to pay is that their reproductive capacity may be permanently impaired. Cryopreservation offers the promise of being able to bank tissue or gametes pre-operatively so that the individual's reproductive capability can be safeguarded. Infertility does not threaten the survival of the individual in the way that, for example, treatment-related cardiac complications might. Infertility does not immediately impair the person's social or intellectual functioning in the manner that damage to the central nervous system might. But infertility can have great personal psychological significance (Dunkel-Schetter and Lobel 1991). Not everyone will want to become a parent but most would like that role to be one of the life-choices open to them (see Chapter 2). Cryopreservation offers a way to keep young patients 'in the game' as it were.

However, the metaphor of buying a ticket or two in life's reproductive lottery glosses over the many risks and uncertainties involved. There will be immediate concerns about the dangers associated with any additional medical procedures such as anaesthesia. Parents may well be sensitive to the emotional impact on their child of being asked to participate in extra treatments when they are already very sick and frightened (as, for example, when a young man might be asked to provide a semen sample – see Chapter 9). In the longer term, questions need to be considered concerning the effectiveness of the storage procedures and the likely success rates of attempts to re-introduce the preserved tissue or gametes. Are miscarriages or birth defects likely to be higher than for 'normally' conceived babies? Where cyropreserved tissue is used in assisted conception treatment, will there be an increased risk of cancer developing for the newborn child or the tissue donors themselves? Good questions all – to which it currently appears harder to give clear answers to some than others (Grundy *et al.* 2001a).

Doctors and patients are faced with difficult treatment choices all the time. It is not often that all the necessary information is available and that an evidently 'right way' forward beckons. Under less optimal circumstances, the effectiveness of treatment decisions needs to be gauged by the manner in which evidence is weighed rather than the correctness of the conclusions reached (i.e. by process rather than outcome criteria). Proponents of 'reasoned choice' models in health care have suggested that there are three essential components of effective decision-taking (Bekker *et al.* 1999):

1.   The decision is based on information relevant to the alternatives and their consequences.

2.   The likelihood and desirability of the consequences are evaluated accurately.

3.   A trade-off between these factors is evident.

At the moment, it appears that the quality of information available to even the best-informed individuals and families is going to be pretty light on convincing statistics of the key likelihood issues of 'prospects of success' and 'risks of medical complications'. The question of desirability raises the thorny matter of exactly whose desires shall have priority in decision-taking. So, at an intellectual level, the criteria required for effective decision-making are already highly demanding.

We also need to consider the circumstances in which this very complicated choice must be made. There may well be a sense of urgency in proceedings. Life-saving treatments cannot be lightly delayed. There will be no opportunity for a change of mind once the decision is made. All families will be highly anxious and quite probably facing a crisis for which they are emotionally unprepared. Although, in legal terms, all adults and some younger people are considered competent to make informed choices on medical matters, it is probably wise to construe this competence as a state rather than a trait. None of us is likely to think too straight when highly stressed and facing an overload of information. Under these circumstances we tend to take cognitive short-cuts (what the psychologists term 'heuristics') to reduce the challenge to a manageable size. A common heuristic employed when patients are confronted by complex medical decisions is to ask health care staff what they would do in the circumstances! Indeed, when decision-making aids have been introduced to enable patients to make more considered, autonomous and 'rational' treatment choices, they are not necessarily appreciated at the time (Bekker, Hewison and Thornton 2003).

In summary, therefore, the decision that we ask individuals and families to make concerning cryopreservation of reproductive tissue and gametes is both highly complex and informationally incomplete. We also ask them to take that decision rapidly and at a time when their collective cognitive functioning is likely to be impoverished. Under these circumstances, we should not be surprised if the choices that are made are heavily subject to external influence.

The family context

As well as considering the complexity of the choices confronting individuals and family members, we should also bear in mind their own history and traditions. Have the parents previously held 'facts of life' conversations with their offspring or are they faced with opening up frank discussions about reproduction for the first time under the most trying of circumstances? If, for example, father and son have talked 'man to man' about sexual matters, did the experience leave both parties happy to return to the subject or was the conversation rapidly foreshortened to avoid further discomfort on either side? Adding embarrassment to an emotional cocktail already brimming with feelings of fear, injustice and uncertainty is unlikely to promote considered decision-taking.

Is there an established problem-solving style in the home to which family members easily revert when under pressure? Will parents with a habit of consulting their children about important family decisions, like where to go on holiday, still be able to retain their democratic principles when their child's survival is at risk? It is perhaps more probable that, confronted by the most powerful reminders of a child's vulnerability, they will find themselves calling more on the dominant stories in our culture about the need for adults to protect incompetent youngsters, rather than prioritizing any responsibility to promote their autonomy (Green, in press). Furthermore, health care workers are also likely to find themselves drawing on the same set of cultural beliefs – as are the young patients themselves. These subtle pressures against the active involvement of young people in medical decision-taking will be considered further in a later section of this chapter.

As well as bearing in mind widely shared cultural assumptions, it is important also to respect the central way in which different cultural beliefs will influence a family's choices about the prospect of cryopreservation of sexual material. For example, Jewish rabbinical teaching is very reluctant to allow masturbation to obtain sperm for testing or insemination (Grazi and Wolowelsky 1995). In Hindu society infertility is highly stigmatizing and any clinical interventions to induce conception may be viewed as an intrusion into the intimacies of the marital relationship (Bharadwaj 2003). Moslem law forbids the use of cryopreserved sperm being used to impregnate a wife after her husband's death (Ahmad 2003). More generally we should anticipate that all religious faiths will have something important to say about the origins of life, and so we should expect that there will be an added spiritual component to the way many families and individuals make sense of their predicament. A sensitivity to these shared cultural beliefs should, nonetheless, not blind us to the varieties of opinion that prevail within, as well as between, communities (Jones and Hunter 1996) (for a wider discussion of culturally sensitive practice, see Chapter 8).

For a significant number of the children and young people, divorce will have been part of their family history. As an indicator, almost one in four children born in 1979 had experienced divorce by the age of 16 (Horton 2004). The goal of enabling family members to come to a 'partnership' decision following parental separation may be further complicated if there has been a subsequent history of troubled communication between the adults. One might speculate that the 'small' matter of the continuation of the family line is likely to arouse strong feelings for divorced parents.

Developmental considerations

When post-pubertal adolescent males are invited to provide semen samples for storage it is probably fair to assume that most will have the cognitive capacity to consent. As the technologies associated with cryopreservation and potential re-implantation of genetic material develop, younger patients will be in a position to benefit from storage of tissue. Should parents then make ethical decisions on their child's behalf or can minors still be included in the choices to be made about their future?

Current advice from the UK Department of Health regarding children and young people's rights to participate in clinical decisions regarding their own treatment is quite explicit (Department of Health 2004a). They should be informed in an age-appropriate manner about exactly the same concerns that adults would have in the same position. What will happen? What are the expected benefits of treatment? Are there any risks involved and how serious are those risks? What might be the consequences of not taking the recommended course of action? Health care staff are encouraged to seek the active consent of all the young people they treat. Although the legal right to refuse treatment is not recognized until the age of 18, good practice is to involve all patients in understanding their illnesses and treatments and to promote shared decision-taking between parents and their children in an age-appropriate manner. Many of these same principles apply to guidance concerning young people's participation in clinical research (Central Office of Research Ethics Committees 2003; Department of Health 2004a). For example, the central point is reiterated that consent without understanding is no consent at all. However, in the research context a young person has greater powers to opt out in their own right. The guidance that 'if you don't like the idea, you can always say no' conveys an unambiguous message.

In practice, however, young people's competence to consent to either medical treatment or participation in clinical research trials does not appear to be widely acknowledged. Although there is some evidence that the culture of paediatric consultations has shifted over recent years to include children in therapeutic conversations more frequently, adult to adult communication continues to dominate proceedings (Tates and Meeuwesen 2001). In the field of paediatric oncology, there is a continuing concern that, particularly at times of crisis, young people may find themselves relegated to 'non-participant status' in consultations between doctors and their families (Young et al. 2003). There is not much reason to suggest that a child's competence to give informed consent to medical procedures is better recognized in the research setting than it is in the clinical setting. Empirical investigation of seven- to nine-year-olds' appreciation of why they had been asked to provide a blood sample for research indicated that most had no real idea but had picked up the sense that the adults seemed to be in favour, so why not? (Ondrusek et al. 1998). The authors of this study conclude that seven-year-olds do not have the cognitive capacity to assent to participate in a research study, though it might also be worth considering whether alternative methods of communication with the children concerned might have resulted in more meaningful agreement. A second study, into children's involvement in leukaemia treatment and research discussions, noted considerable variability in the degree to which clinicians included young people in consultations regarding their participation in a clinical trial (Olechnowicz *et al.* 2002). Although there was some suggestion from the results that the young person's involvement increased with age, the predominant pattern was again adult-to-adult communication. Indeed, the more questions parents posed of the physician, the less likely was s/he to direct subsequent questions towards the young patient.

A further complication for parents is the challenge of respecting the views that their child is currently able to express, while simultaneously trying to imagine the opinion that the same child might hold at some time in the future (McCall Smith 2004). Follow-up studies of young men whose fertility has been compromised by treatment for childhood cancer (Green, Galvin and Horne 2003) have reported not only considerable differences between individuals in the personal significance they attach to the prospect of fathering children but also how dramatically the strength of these feelings can vary over time (depending, for example, on the status of their romantic relationships). A concerned mother may well be prepared to over-rule a child's wish not to receive a painful injection because, as a responsible parent, she appreciates that the long-term benefits of medical treatment will outweigh the short-term discomfort the child will experience. She is unlikely, however, to find it so straightforward to strike an optimal balance between immediate preferences and future possibilities when faced with the prospect of tissue storage. Do we decide against putting further pressure on a sick and scared child or do we deny the child an opportunity to decide for themselves and in their own time whether they want to keep their reproductive options open in this way?

Then what?

There is a consensus within the field of medical ethics that informed consent should be understood as a continuing process rather than a one-off decision captured forever by a signature on a form (Royal College of Physicians 1996). Consider the way that time might alter the manner in which a decision to preserve tissue or gametes might be perceived by the parties involved. Inevitably, the child or young person themselves will become increasingly able to grasp the complexities of their circumstance as they grow older. With experience, their sexual preferences and ambitions will become more established. Ongoing medical research will provide more and better information on the viability of the whole cryopreservation strategy. Will storage methods prove to be safe and effective? How will the evidence concerning any increase in the probability of recurring disease stack up? The legislative scene may also change to keep track of developing medical technology. And, of course, a proportion of those who stored their material will, sadly, not survive to adulthood.

Some young cancer survivors can reach adulthood without having been properly informed about the impact that medical treatment has had on their reproductive potential (Green et al. 2003). They are not generally pleased to have been kept in this state of ignorance. It would be equally inappropriate for childhood cancer survivors to grow up unaware that samples of reproductive tissue have been stored on their behalf. What they and others similarly affected should be told, when and by whom are questions for debate and empirical investigation. That this conversation should take place seems indisputable. Furthermore, this should be the first of a series of ongoing communications on the topic. We expect any bank that looks after our money and valuables to keep us regularly updated on the status of our investments. We might also seek specialist advice if our circumstances change and we wish our lives to take new directions. This financial metaphor can be pushed too far, but the analogy is helpful in emphasizing the rights of the consumer and the quality of the ongoing service s/he can reasonably expect from the Health Service. It also acts as a reminder that the purpose of the whole enterprise is to allow the tissue or gametes provider him or herself to maintain the possibility of becoming the genetic parent of their own child. If they die or elect not to become a parent, what should become of the stored material? There is an attractive ethical clarity in adopting the position that, unless the person has given an explicit direction to the contrary, the tissue or gamete should be destroyed.

No doubt such material could be put to significant use in research, but the medical establishment in the UK ought to have been thoroughly sensitized to the risks involved in retaining any remains of deceased children's bodies without the unambiguous permission of the bereaved family (House of Commons 2001). The extended legal debate over Diane Blood's wish to use her husband's cryopreserved sperm to have another child after his death would, no doubt, have been greatly simplified if Stephen Blood had been able to indicate his own opinions about this route to posthumous parenthood (HFEA 1996).

Conclusion

In this chapter we have set out the legal framework surrounding cryopreservation of reproductive material in one jurisdiction, the UK. We have used this as a backdrop to consider the considerable complexities attached to the decision-making about whether or not to store and to its aftermath. Scientific advances bring with them social, emotional and ethical challenges that are rarely easy to unscramble – and perhaps there are none more so than those to be negotiated when seeking to preserve the potential for future life at the same time as coping with a threat to mortality in the present.

Note

1 This Act does not confer any inheritance or nationality rights on to any children conceived posthumously.

Part Three

Personal Experiences of Living with Health Conditions and Disability and the Impact on Sexuality and Fertility

8

Disability, Chronic Illness, Fertility and Minority Ethnic Young People
Making Sense of Identity, Diversity and Difference

Karl Atkin, Amanda Rodney and Francine Cheater

Introduction

This chapter is a little different from others in this volume. It has a broader scope. Such a focus, however, makes a great deal of sense. There is little discussion and much less research exploring ethnicity and fertility (Culley *et al.* 2004; National Institute for Clinical Excellence 2004). This is perhaps not surprising and represents a more general problem: research rarely responds to the multi-ethnic nature of developed countries, while policy and practice struggle to engage with minority ethnic populations (Atkin 2004). At best this means the perspectives and needs as defined by minority ethnic people and their families do not adequately inform the priorities of public services (Social Services Inspectorate 2000). At worst it means that policy and practice are informed by racist myths and stereotypes (Ahmad 2000).

This is why, when trying to understand a particular issue such as growing up with fertility difficulties, we need to begin by exploring the context in which we come to make sense of ideas such as diversity, difference and disadvantage (Mason 2000). This provides an initial framework in which to understand the experience of young people and their families as they negotiate transitions to adulthood (Karslen and Nazroo 2002). It also ensures that any future debates about fertility and ethnicity are not only appropriately contextualized with ongoing theoretical debates but also able to make use of, and develop, transferable empirical insights gained from the more general literature.

Taking this as our starting point, this chapter offers an agenda for future engagement for those wishing to explore fertility, sexuality and ethnicity in which broader concepts such as citizenship, social justice and identity assume prominence. In adopting such a position our aim is not to offer 'essentialized' cultural accounts that treat minority ethnic populations as the 'other'. Our chapter, therefore, will not offer neat prescriptive cultural descriptions that purport to explain 'ethnicity' and fertility. Not everything can be reduced to culture. Our concern is to offer a broader discussion that appropriately contextualizes diversity and difference in a way that enables fertility policy, practice and research to engage with, and understand, minority ethnic populations without recourse to simplistic explanations and naive solutions that perpetuate disadvantage and discrimination.

We begin with an account of institutional racism – a concept that has assumed recent legitimacy in explaining disadvantage and discrimination. We then specifically explore what is meant by diversity and difference and end by reflecting on the importance of using evidence to improve outcomes. Throughout the chapter we draw out differences and similarities between the experience of minority ethnic people and the dominant ethnic population and introduce relevant empirical examples.

Young people, citizenship and disadvantage: understanding fertility and ethnicity

We start by exploring how received ideas of legitimacy and interpretation inform engagement with minority ethnic people who have fertility problems. 'Institutional racism' has recently become a popular explanation for the inability of services to respond to the needs of an ethnically diverse society. In the UK context this can be attributed directly to the Macpherson Enquiry (1999) into the death of Steven Lawrence.[1] Macpherson provided the term with moral authority, which found legal expression with the introduction, in April 2001, of amendments to the 1976 Race Relations Act. These made statutory agencies – including health and social care agencies – responsible for promoting equal opportunities and identifying and tackling institutional racism within their organizations (see Commission for Racial Equality 2003).

Despite recent interest, institutional racism is not a new idea. The concept was first introduced over 20 years ago (Glasgow 1980). Since then, institutional racism has emerged as an extremely helpful and productive idea in making sense of inequalities as well as inappropriate and inaccessible health and social care provision (Law 1996). It is this analytical legitimacy and the extent to which it captures the essence of ethnic discrimination that now concern us. Making sense of this represents an important starting point in developing fertility support that is sensitive to the needs of minority ethnic populations.

At its most straightforward, institutional racism is often called camouflaged racism, meaning that it is not immediately obvious but embedded in the taken-for-granted assumptions informing organization practices (Mason 2000). It occurs when the policies of an institution lead to discriminatory outcomes for minority ethnic populations, irrespective of the motives of individual employees of that institution. Institutional racism is the uncritical application of policies and procedures that ignore or misrepresent the needs of an ethnically diverse society (Butt and Mirza 1996).

There is evidence that fertility services embody many aspects of institutionally racist practices (see for example Culley *et al.* 2004; Katbamna, Bhakta and Parker 2000; Schmid *et al.* 2004). Minority ethnic patients struggle to gain appropriate language support, have to engage with practitioners who make little concession to possible cultural differences in how the experience of fertility is interpreted and are subject to ill-informed assumptions about their family relationships and reproductive practices. In developing its relevance to our discussion we need, however, to explore the concept of institutional racism further. To this extent, two general and inter-related themes help explain why current health and social care is ill-equipped to respond to cultural differences and why practitioners find it difficult to understand the lifestyles, social customs and religious practices of minority ethnic people.

Ignoring need

First, potential differences in need between minority ethnic people and the general population are often disregarded because there is an underlying assumption that policies, procedures and practices are equally appropriate for everyone (Ahmad 2000). Such practices, by default, favour the majority White population who come to represent the 'norm' around which service delivery becomes organized (Law 1996). Service users, for example, are assumed to have Western attitudes, priorities, expectations and values, to act according to Western ways, to speak English and to understand the organization of public services (Parekh 2000).

The inability of the NHS to provide adequate support for those whose first language is not English is the most obvious example of this and has particular implications for fertility services where offering detailed information to young people and their families is essential in ensuring that they can exercise appropriate choices (Culley *et al.* 2004). Language is not the only barrier to successful communication. Nonetheless, it is helpful to explore the issue in detail as it represents an important illustration of how health care agencies struggle to engage with difference and diversity and the consequences of this failure for minority ethnic populations.

In the first instance, interpreters are often in short supply (Association of London Government 2000). When a person cannot speak English, family members are sometimes used as interpreters. Although acceptable to some people, others object to the practice (Robinson 2001). In some cases, children and young people are required to act as interpreters of complex medical information about fertility and sexuality; often about sensitive or potentially embarrassing issues (Schmid *et al.* 2004). Young people have pointed to the problems they face in simultaneously translating distressing information to their parents – either about themselves or their siblings – and coming to terms with it themselves (Bhakta, Katbamna and Parker 2000). Young people have also spoken of difficulties in deciding how much they should tell their non-English-speaking parents: they want to 'protect them' from information deemed upsetting. This, however, often leaves non-English-using parents or family members without important information; information vital for understanding and coping as well as for deciding what course of action to take (Atkin 2004).

Difficulties still occur when interpreters are used (Robinson 2001). Most interpreters, for example, face difficulties in interpreting specific clinical information and procedures, sometimes with unfortunate consequences. In Punjabi, for instance, the phrase 'born with the condition' can become confused with 'genetic condition' and Atkin (2004) cites an example of a family who did not realize until the birth of their third thalassaemic child that the condition was a recessive genetic disorder. Anionwu and Atkin (2001) mention similar examples in which the possible fertility difficulties associated with bone marrow transplants are poorly explained to South Asian families because of the difficulties of finding English terms that have the same conceptual equivalence in Punjabi and Urdu. These difficulties mean that young people and their families can often gain misleading and erroneous information about their fertility options (see Culley *et al.* 2004 for a discussion of the broader implications of this).

Families also point to the problems of communicating through a third party (Anionwu and Atkin 2001). This, they felt, made it difficult to ask questions and more generally to take part in a discussion with health professionals. Many practitioners, for their part, share these concerns (Phelan and Parkman 1995) as well as question their own competence in working with interpreters (Ali, Neal and Atkin 2003). It is rare for practitioners to have been trained in the use of interpreters and this perhaps goes some way to explain their unease with the process (Phelan and Parkman 1995). Practitioners often feel they convey little more than superficial information, which rarely does justice to the complexity of the issues they are trying to convey (see Atkin 2004).

The difficulties of providing adequate language support create barriers to effective communication and make it difficult to respond to the care needs of some minority ethnic populations. The problems of language, however, should be seen in perspective (Modood, Betthould and Lakey 1997). There is an unfortunate history of conceptualizing language difficulties as the major difficulty facing public organizations as they struggle to engage with minority ethnic populations. Language problems are simply one of many difficulties (Bradby 2003). Even if there were resources for an expansion of interpreting provision and greater translation of information into different languages, many fundamental problems would still remain. Barriers to communication are more than language-specific and evoke cultural differences, particularly since ethnic and cultural misunderstandings, myths and stereotypes can undermine the communication process (Johnson 1999; Netto *et al.* 2001). Making sense of this introduces our second theme.

Misrepresenting need
When difference is recognized, it is often done in such a way as to misrepresent the health care needs of minority ethnic populations. There are several ways in which this is done. Sometimes it is the consequence of ill-informed views about the cause of problems presented by minority ethnic populations. Health and social agencies, for example, often identify minority ethnic health and social 'problems' as arising from 'pathological' cultural practices (see Ahmad, Atkin and Jones 2002; Bowler 1993; Mir and Tovey

2003). There is a history of defining health problems faced by South Asian and African-Caribbean populations in terms of cultural deficits, where a shift towards a 'Western' lifestyle is offered as a solution to their problems. Examples include discussion on maternity and child health, diet and rickets (see Mason 2000). Such views become embedded in the views of front-line practitioners working in health and social services; minority ethnic people become seen as 'a problem' (Ahmad 2000). Practitioners working in local authorities often list South Asian people as 'high risk' clients, 'uncooperative' and 'difficult to work with'. Similarly, evidence suggests that racism within the NHS affects minority ethnic people, with common stereotypes portraying them as 'calling out doctors unnecessarily', 'being trivial complainers', and 'time wasters'. These attitudes can, of course, deprive minority ethnic people of their rights to services (see Atkin 2004 for a review of the literature).

There is evidence that such assumptions are not uncommon in fertility services, which raises the possibility that minority ethnic populations can become blamed for their difficulties (see Culley *et al.* 2004; Schmid *et al.* 2004). A more detailed empirical example, with potential lessons for those developing work around fertility and ethnicity, will illustrate this further and concerns how 'poor childhood health' among South Asian families becomes attributed to consanguineous (related by blood) marriages (see Ahmad, Atkin and Chamba 2000 for a review of the evidence). A young person's fertility problems can easily become bound up in such discussions. Given the pervasive nature of such assumptions, it might become easy to associate a child's infertility with consanguineous marriage between his or her parents.

The relationship between consanguineous marriage and poor health is, of course, complex. In some cases, marrying a first cousin can increase a family's risk of having a disabled or chronically ill child, especially if there is a history of certain conditions in the extended family. First cousin marriage, however, is not the only cause of disability or chronic illness in Pakistani or Bangladeshi families and there is good evidence to suggest that its influence has been over-emphasized. Such an association, however, is well embedded in professional practices. Ahmad *et al.* (2000) cite the case of a couple who had recently had a child with thalassaemia (a recessively inherited blood disorder, which is transmitted in the same way as sickle cell disorders and cystic fibrosis). The health professionals involved insisted that the couple were first cousins, when they were not.[2] Such assumptions not only carry an implicit (and misleading) criticism of Asian cultural practices, they also misrepresent the origins of ill health and therefore lead to misguided policy approaches that can serve to alienate families. The preoccupation with consanguineous marriage means other important explanations – such as poverty, poor maternal health, inappropriate housing, or inadequate service support – are rarely mentioned.

At other times, inappropriate myths and stereotypes, although purporting to explain the behaviour and beliefs of minority ethnic populations, do little more than misrepresent their experience (see Parekh 2000 for a discussion of these issues). African-Caribbean people's experience of pain relief illustrates this (Allenye and Thomas 1994). African-Caribbean young people often complain about the poor treatment of pain when they are on hospital wards (see Anionwu and Atkin 2001). Some of the assumptions held by ward staff help to explain this. A common myth among doctors and nurses is that African-Caribbean people exaggerate their pain because they have lower pain thresholds. Some doctors and nurses also believe that African-Caribbean people are more prone to become addicted to powerful pain killers than other ethnic populations and therefore withhold treatment (Anionwu and Atkin 2001; Schechter, Berrien and Katz 1988). There is, of course, no scientific basis for such assumptions, but they are used by health care agencies as a reason for not meeting the care needs of African-Caribbean people.

Ironically, some of the problems associated with myths and stereotypes occur because authors want to be helpful and to provide explanations that enable professionals to respond to the needs of a multi-ethnic society. Introductory notes on minority ethnic communities that are present in most training materials for service practitioners often follow this pattern. Examples adopting such approaches are emerging in the literature on fertility. Muslim families' responses to their children's fertility problems, for instance, cannot be summarized in a couple of pages as there is no one Muslim response to fertility problems. Diversity is the key. Such explanations tend to present static and one-dimensional views of cultural norms and values, are devoid of context and allow no room for individual interpretation (Atkin 2004). They also create the illusion that they offer a solution to an extremely complex situation (Chattoo and Ahmad 2004).

Identity, diversity and difference: young people's experience of fertility difficulties

Understanding barriers to providing responsive and equitable service provision for minority ethnic populations suggests further themes relevant to our debate. Ethnicity is a notoriously difficult concept to define and conceptual confusion sometimes occurs (Bradby 2003). In some ways, the multi-faceted nature in which we have come to understand 'ethnicity' has advantages as we attempt to tackle disadvantages and discrimination (Chattoo, Atkin and McNeish 2004). If nothing else, it reminds us of the complex and shifting nature of ethnicity, as it comes to embody language, religion, culture, nationality and a shared heritage (Ahmad *et al.* 2002). Ethnicity is also increasingly seen as a political symbol, defining not just exclusion by a powerful majority but also a source of pride and belonging that enables minority ethnic populations to celebrate their difference (Parekh 2000; Werbner 1997).

Policy and practice, however, still associate 'ethnicity' with the 'other' and, by failing to engage with the relationship between ethnicity, socio-economic status, age and gender, can obscure fundamental similarities as well as differences among populations (see, for example, Chamba *et al.* 1999; Nazroo 1997; Smaje and Field 1997). We now explore this in greater detail and draw out the specific implications of these debates for making sense of young people's experience of fertility problems. As a start, we need to be aware of how fertility difficulties relate to young people's broader conception of who they are. This requires understanding them as 'young people' rather than 'young people with fertility problems'. Exploring identity is fundamental to this.

Identity, ethnicity, young people and their families

How can we make sense of identity, which often evokes abstract and esoteric debates, in a way relevant to our discussion? In the first instance, when making sense of a young person's fertility problems, we need to conceptualize a young person's relationship with their parents and significant others, define their sense of intergenerational notions of rights, responsibilities and duty, discuss how ethnicity and culture are negotiated as lived experiences, and identify how gender, social class, migration history and socio-economic position of the family mediate family values. Present debates about young people, however, are rarely framed in this way and this creates difficulties when trying to understand a young person's response to fertility difficulties.

There is, for example, little sociological literature on young people within the context of their family life and more on the structural features of class and youth as a category. This occurs irrespective of ethnicity. Young people are often perceived as subjects of observation and surveillance and this emphasizes problems and potential conflict (Brannen *et al.* 1994). We also know little about the interface between cultural and legal notions of childhood and transitions to adult status (Punch 2003). Given that concepts central to our ideas of childhood, such as 'independence', vary between cultures and within communities, previous accounts can reflect ethnocentric perspectives (Katz 2002; Morrow 1998). The idea of 'independent living' for disabled young people, for instance, can acquire different meanings for South Asian families. From a Western perspective, independent living assumes living away from the parental home. For some South Asian young people, independent living can be achieved within their family home and does not necessarily require them to leave (Hussain, Atkin and Ahmad 2002).

Furthermore, the broader literature on family obligations, identity and social change rarely engages with the experience of minority ethnic families and, when it does, it focuses on issues such as migration, settlement patterns, economic survival and racism (see Finch and Mason 1993; Qureshi and Walker 1989). This provides for a skewed debate and, in the absence of sound, comparative research, policy-makers and practitioners are faced with opposing stereotypes. On one hand there are assumptions about uniquely virtuous, supportive, extended minority ethnic families caring for their own (Bhakta *et al.* 2000). At the same time, social policy and lay discourses often assume social change to be a consequence of the process of acculturation or adoption of the values of the 'host society' by the younger generation. This is perceived to result in an inevitable conflict of values between the older and younger generation or, at worst, a generation of estranged young people trapped between cultures (see Ahmad 1996 for a review). Research findings, however, do not support such a view and although differences in values between generations do occur, there is also a great deal of continuity (see Chattoo *et al.* 2004; Hussain *et al.* 2002).

The idea that identities are situational and flexible is, of course, not new (Papastergiadis 1982). Being a young person, generational relations, social class, gender, sexuality, ethnicity and religion, for example, represent important identifications. The inter-relationship between these identifications are complex and intimately connected to questions of power, structure and history (Ahmad *et al.* 2002). This is the extent to which 'local cultures and values' impact on people's experience of fertility (Nizalova 2000), particularly since sexuality and gender identities become intimately bound up with fertility. This in turn illustrates why we should guard against allowing ill-informed, generalized cultural stereotypes to inform the development of service support. What then are the implications of this for policy and practice?

Understanding ethnicity and diversity

We need to accept that, in some ways, minority ethnic populations may not be all that different from the general population. The challenge is to know when ethnicity does make a difference and mediate a person's experience and when it does not. This challenge has particular relevance for this chapter where evidence suggests ethnicity is one variable among many in explaining people's response to fertility. Education and socio-economic background can sometimes be as important as a person's ethnic origin (Burr and Bean 1996; Gangadharan 2001; Rindfuss, Morgan and Offutt 1996; Ventura 1995). When looking at differences between Latinos and Anglo women in North America, Chavez (2004) concluded that ethnic differences were insignificant: age, education and marital status were more relevant in making sense of their experience of fertility. There is no reason to think that these findings do not apply at least in part to young people's experience.

South Asian parents' and young people's discussions about fertility following bone marrow transplantation in thalassaemia further illustrate the importance of conceptualizing ethnicity within this broader context (see Anionwu and Atkin 2001). Several years after the event, parents and young people often complain that they were not informed about the possible effects on fertility following bone marrow transplantation. Research, however, suggests that they were informed but at the time chose to focus on the prospect of 'cure' rather than the long-term consequences of the treatment. This is perhaps understandable, particularly since bone marrow transplantation occurs at a young age when fertility may not always be uppermost in a parent's mind. Such a response, however, occurs irrespective of ethnicity and seems to be a feature of bone marrow transplantation.

Ethnicity, therefore, does not always equate with difference. Similarly, not every problem or difficulty a person encounters as they attempt to gain access to appropriate service delivery can be attributed to his or her ethnic background. Socio-economic status, age and gender may be as important as ethnicity in making sense of a person's health and social care needs (Nazroo 1997). By improving services generally we can often improve support for minority ethnic populations.

Disability, chronic illness and identity

Up to now we have discussed identity within the broader context of ethnicity, diversity and difference. There has been, however, an important theme missing from our discussion. Many of the issues raised by more specific discussions about ethnicity, chronic illness and disability have relevance to emerging discourses on fertility and ethnicity. Debates about identity are complex but are perhaps more so for disabled or chronically ill people from minority ethnic groups. Young people may wish to identify with the religious and cultural values of their family as well as with those of the more Western-orientated wider society in which they live. The experience of disability in which they are struggling to reconcile the inability of the wider society to accommodate difference, while maintaining a positive identity, further complicates the situation (Oliver 1996).

The past 20 years have seen a shift in how disability is perceived in Western societies. The medical model, with its emphasis on rehabilitation and sense of personal tragedy, has been challenged by a more social model in which disability is seen in relation to the attitudes and barriers imposed by an unjust society (Oliver 1996). Disability thus becomes a social issue in which systematic discrimination not only leads to loss of independence and choice for disabled people but also excludes them from activities and roles taken for granted by the majority of the population (Corker and French 1998). This powerful critique, by showing that many of the disadvantages faced by disabled people result from wider society's inability to accommodate difference, has informed disabled people's political struggle for a positive identity. Autonomy, inclusion, control of resources, independent living and claims to equal citizenship emerge as important symbols in the positive re-framing of disability (Swain *et al.* 2004).

Despite its considerable and valuable role in asserting the rights of disabled people, the disability movement itself has been criticized for not recognizing diversity (Stuart 1996). Struggles to maintain a positive self-identity while engaging with negative public assumptions about disability and social disadvantage occur, of course, irrespective of ethnicity (see Oliver

1996). Disability, however, can only be understood against what is considered as 'normal' for someone of that particular age, gender, social class and ethnic and religious background (Ahmad 2000). Normalcy is not a given universal and needs to be seen in its social and cultural context. Consequently, as we have seen, independence and autonomy may not have the same meaning among different social groups (Hussain *et al.* 2002).

A more specific example illustrates this further and concerns the choice of young South Asian disabled people's marriage partners, particularly since such choices occur in relation to a preference for negotiated marriages among some South Asian communities. Since a sense of 'spoiled identity' underpins some of their experiences, important parallels emerge relevant to debates about fertility. South Asian disabled people express various concerns about marriage and about perceptions of their suitability as marriage partners, which reflect their more general sense of disadvantage as disabled people (see Hussain *et al.* 2002). Despite these concerns, Hussain *et al.* (2002) note that marriage still remained important to young disabled people and their families and reflected the cultural importance of marriage in South Asian communities. Impairment, however, did mediate marriage negotiations and differences did emerge between the expectations of the disabled young person and their non-disabled siblings. Disabled young people often felt that they had to accept 'second best' and believed that their brothers and sisters were more likely to find suitable partners. Perhaps for these reasons, parents and disabled young people felt it was easier to bring marriage partners from overseas rather than try to find marriage partners in the UK. Overseas partners were seen as having lower expectations and to be more willing to come to the UK, particularly since there was the additional opportunity of settling in the UK.

Achieving change and improving outcomes: developing successful fertility services

The final discursive practice with which we need to engage embodies another fundamental key tension. The critical emphasis of current literature on ethnicity, health and social care is perhaps understandable and has successfully highlighted the negative consequences of racism, marginalization and unequal treatment (Mason 2000). Policy and practice, however, have been less successful in translating these insights into improvements in service delivery (Atkin 2004). Consequently, practitioners often feel overwhelmed about providing care for people from diverse cultural and linguistic back-grounds (Qureshi, Berridge and Wenman 2000). They are increasingly burdened by the volume of evidence reminding them of their failure to pro-vide accessible and appropriate care and are regularly presented with advice offering little more than bland statements emphasizing the importance of responding to cultural diversity and tackling discrimination, while provid-ing no tangible framework with which to improve care (see Atkin 2004). Minority ethnic populations, for their part, are becoming increasingly disil-lusioned about contributing to research on which such guidance is based, without seeing any tangible improvements in service delivery (Mir and Nocon 2002).

Offering an analysis of the problems facing minority ethnic populations is one thing; doing something about them is another. Those providing fer-tility services for minority ethnic populations can learn valuable lessons from previous mistakes. More needs to be understood, for example, about what constitutes good practice and how such practice can be implemented effectively, sustained in the longer term and replicated in other localities. More research outlining the difficulties facing minority ethnic populations is perhaps unhelpful. Research needs to re-focus its attention on under-standing how services can best meet the needs of minority ethnic populations, by exploring how services are delivered and suggesting ways of how they can be improved. As well as defining problems, our growing evidence base must also offer potential solutions. Without such a commitment to change, ser-vice initiatives are not only in danger of wasting valuable public resources but are also in jeopardy of becoming little more than token gestures leading to increasing estrangement among minority ethnic populations.

Conclusion

Despite gradual improvement and an increasing awareness of the complex nature of culturally sensitive provision, health and social care providers experience difficulties in meeting the care needs of various minority ethnic populations. Debates about ethnicity, sexuality and fertility, including for those making the transition to adulthood, reflect these problems. The lack of research and informed policy discussion, however, makes it difficult for us to offer a specific conclusion. Nonetheless, we are able to contextualize and utilize insights from broader debates, which can enable those with an interest in fertility and ethnicity to develop a greater understanding of the subject.

There is little doubt that a person's ethnic background is likely to have a considerable impact on their relationship to fertility services (Culley *et al.* 2004). Services have struggled to offer appropriate and accessible care to minority ethnic populations. Institutional racism is a useful concept in explaining such disadvantage and the evidence offers many instances where professional assumptions and organizational practices reduce minority ethnic populations to monolithic, homogeneous communities defined by their ethnicity, religion or culture, with little reflection on differences within and similarities across communities. Such a preoccupation also deflects attention away from structural issues of inequality and forms of institutional cultures and racism that sustain these inequalities (Gunaratnam 1997).

Understanding ethnicity, however, also embodies 'being' and this is where a person's sense of cultural identity may become meaningful. Young people emerge as active social agents who create and negotiate values and meanings within the context of their social identity. Continuity and change represent the creative dynamic at the heart of who these young people are. Western values are considered alongside – and not instead of – their parents' values: it is rarely a question of forsaking one claim for another. Understanding the complexity of the family life of minority ethnic communities (as with any community) is another essential component in developing successful provision.

Fertility policy and practice need to reflect such diversity and not assume that Western ideas, values and priorities have the same relevance for all minority ethnic people and their families. In particular, service provision needs to become more sensitive to the cultural and religious values held by young people and their families and to recognize how these interact with the experience of fertility (see Payne 2004 and Smallwood and Jefferies 2003 for the implications of this for fertility services). At the same time, it must be recognized that ethnicity might not be the only explanation of difference and disadvantage.

To conclude, our account suggests that successful policy and practice in developing fertility support need to engage with two distinct aspects of welfare provision. First, research, policy and practice need to provide a clear insight into how current discursive practices engage with the experience of minority ethnic populations and to reconcile this with the narratives of young people and their families. This begins to provide an initial evidence base and critical insight. Second, when discussing these issues, policy and practice have to have a commitment to change. Focusing on the needs of minority ethnic populations is not the same as responding to those needs. This, however, requires a broader cultural shift in how service providers engage with minority ethnic populations.

Notes

1 Stephen Lawrence, an African-Caribbean young man, was murdered by White racists in London, UK. The Metropolitan Police did not initially take the crime seriously and Macpherson attributed this to institutionally racist practices.
2 Interestingly, sickle cell disorders and cystic fibrosis, recessive conditions that largely occur in different ethnic groups, are not attributed to consanguineous marriage.

9.

The Sting in the Tail
Teenagers Coping with Sperm Banking Following a Cancer Diagnosis

Marilyn Crawshaw[1]

Introduction

The provision of fertility preservation services through sperm banking to young men under the age of majority facing treatment for cancer and other potentially sterilizing health conditions or treatments is a relatively new service throughout the world. In the UK it is regulated through the Human Fertilisation and Embryology Act 1990 (HFE Act) under the auspices of the Human Fertilisation & Embryology Authority (HFEA). Although the HFE Act was implemented as recently as 1991, such is the pace of change in this field of medical science that few minors were banking at that time and no special provision was made for them either in services or in consent requirements. This has left the unique situation whereby only the young men themselves can consent to semen storage and there can be no substituted consent by proxies, including parents (HFE Act Schedule 3). Where mature gametes are present, the young men therefore must be deemed competent to use fertility preservation services. Decisions have to be made and acted on between diagnosis and commencement of treatment, when young men (some as young as 13) and their parents are in a state of shock. (For a fuller discussion of the legal and ethical issues, see Chapter 7.)

Researchers and practitioners have suggested that the impact of a cancer diagnosis during the teenage years brings unique pressures, coming as it does during the demanding emotional and social pressures of moving towards adulthood (Neville 1998; Roberts, Turney and Knowles 1998; Schover 1997). The onset of cancer typically heightens the young person's dependency on their family, thus stalling or even reversing any trend to spend more time away from the family unit and with peers. Research also suggests that teenagers' primary sources of knowledge about sexuality and fertility are teachers and friends (see Chapter 3) and these too may be affected.

Professionals' concerns about their knowledge and skills base in providing an age-appropriate fertility preservation service and the associated ethical issues have been noted (Bahadur *et al.* 2001; Crawshaw *et al.* 2004; Multi-disciplinary Working Group 2003; Schover *et al.* 2002).

The absence of any systematic collection and analysis of the experiences of those directly involved is a significant drawback to service development.

Background to the study

Given the lack of existing research and the sensitive nature of the subject, it was agreed that a pilot study should be undertaken initially, funded by the UK National Health Service. As part of that study, 22 interviews were held with a range of professionals from paediatric oncology and reproductive medicine, nursing, reproductive science and social work, primarily from two regional paediatric oncology centres and three assisted conception units that had sperm banks in the North of England.

These interviews established the professionals' understanding of the processes in their local fertility preservation service and identified any concerns about its delivery. This, together with findings from the literature, served the purpose of orienting the researchers to local and national services and issues, and identifying areas on which professionals would welcome feedback (a crucial factor in effecting service change) (Crawshaw *et al.* 2003, 2004).

National postal surveys of all UK assisted conception units and regional paediatric oncology centres were also undertaken to document common practices, areas of variance and professional issues (Crawshaw *et al.* 2003; Glaser *et al.* 2004).

Methodology

Local Research Ethics Committees' approval was obtained.

Interviews

Single interviews were undertaken that focused on the young men's and parents' retrospective perceptions of the content and style of communication within the family and with professionals surrounding the decision-making about, and management of, sperm storage following a diagnosis of cancer. A qualitative approach was used to allow respondents to raise issues pertinent to them (Robson 1998). Prompts were made either for clarification or when respondents appeared to have completed their narrative. Towards the end, the researcher invited comment on areas not spontaneously covered using a topic guide. Permission was given for all interviews to be taped and transcribed.

Framework analysis (Ritchie and Spencer 1994) was used to analyse the interview data. Two researchers, including the one who conducted the interviews, separately read and analysed the transcripts to identify themes, then a final framework was reached through discussion between the researchers. Respondents were sent summaries of the analysis before the full report was written in order to test the researchers' interpretations against the research participants' perceptions. Finally, findings from the interviews with professionals, the young men and their parents were compared.

Sample

Potential recruits who were under 18 (the age of consent in England) and post-Tanner Stage 2^2 at diagnosis were approached by paediatric oncology staff when they were not undergoing intensive treatment. Their involvement was discussed with their parents/carers where appropriate (and always if they were under 16). Parents were invited to be interviewed, with their sons' permission.

Due to high levels of relapse in the potential sample, only nine young men were approached. Of these, seven young men and five sets of parents agreed to participate. Five young men were interviewed alone while two opted to have a parent present.

There was a diversity among the young men according to age (14 to 17 at diagnosis and 16 to 20 at interview); ethnicity (six White, one Asian); disability (one had a prior physical disability and at least one had learning difficulties); living situation (with a single parent [1], both parents [3], another family member [1] and alone [2]); and employment situation (in education

[3], full time employment [2], unemployed/on sick leave [2]) and cancer type. Two parents were lone parents; three were from two-parent families.

To maintain confidentiality, their situation is not generally referred to. The analysis did not reveal differences related to specific situations. Quotes are drawn from all respondents.

Findings

Despite the small numbers being interviewed, their experiences are recounted here as they echoed or illustrated some of the concerns expressed in other parts of the study – for example those around the consent process, including the impact of the need for urgency even though there were already significant levels of stress for all around the cancer diagnosis. Also of concern was the uncertainty among service providers about the format and manner in which to provide relevant information. The young men and their parents offer helpful insights into this. Finally, the service providers gave hints that they did not know whether or not sperm banking was important to such young men – the voices heard here leave one in no doubt about its importance for many.

All the young men interviewed were offered sperm storage. Of the three who refused, one remained sure of his decision but two had some regrets. On the whole, all had high levels of recall about this aspect of their cancer experience though, of course, this is not necessarily the same as high levels of accuracy of factual detail. There were very few discrepancies between the young men's and parents' accounts. The young men, including those who did not go on to bank, were generally able to express their feelings and to talk reflectively about their experiences, which is of note given the diversity of their backgrounds. They appeared to welcome the opportunity to talk about their experience, seek information and influence future practice. Several said this was the first time that they had explored the area of fertility in such a focused way. Interviews with both parents and sons typically ran in excess of an hour.

Several key themes emerged about the young men's experiences and those of their parents:

- the importance of having choices
- the pressure of decision-making and consenting
- the need for information

- the significance of fertility preservation
- the importance of communication with professionals and others.

The importance of having choices

All the young men welcomed the opportunity to consider banking, including those who decided against storage. All discussed their decision, albeit in varying amounts, with at least one parent, usually the mother. Only one discussed it with friends as he had a particularly close pre-existing friendship group. The importance of dialogue with parents was stressed, as were the potential or actual difficulties where there was no history of openness about sexuality, fertility or relationship issues.

Despite overwhelming concern for their sons' survival and, for some, lack of experience in talking about such intimate matters, parents were on the whole able actively to give time and attention to help them make the decision. There was a strong sense on both sides that the final decision appropriately rested with the young men even though both were aware of their youth, state of shock, and feelings of embarrassment:

> And I sat him down and I says […] it's up to you at the end of the day what you do… Now I know it's going to be really horrible and you don't want me to know about this, but if you don't do this you'll never ever have a chance to have a baby… I had to try and get it through to him that it was his only chance of really having his own baby. (Mother)

However, level of parental involvement did not appear to be the single influential factor in decision-making. Although neither of the two with some regrets had been able to discuss it in depth with their parents, both felt that other factors were in fact more influential – one was physically unable to try to bank; the other referred to embarrassment and the timing of being asked as barriers.

The experience of being offered the service varied. Few felt that they had much choice over its timing but accepted the need for it to be raised soon after diagnosis. Within that constraint, two young men felt it could have been addressed more quickly, one would have liked someone to talk to while waiting to bank and one felt he had to wait too long to bank and believed that this unnecessarily (and stressfully) delayed the start of treatment.

Only a minority of the young men remembered having any choice about whether or not to have a parent present when the subject was raised, regardless of age. The two (aged 14 and 16 respectively at diagnosis) who had a choice felt content with the one they made. For two others, the lack of choice was not an issue – one (aged 17 at diagnosis) was alone when it was raised, the other (aged 16 at diagnosis) was with both parents. For others, lack of choice led to difficulties that could have been avoided. For example, one was accompanied by his mother, with whom he had a close relationship, and his estranged father. The consultant assumed (wrongly) that it was preferable only to have the father present and asked the mother to leave. The mother was left to mend a difficult reaction by her son at the same time as re-engaging him in the decision to be made.

Parents generally felt the introduction of fertility preservation had been done well but also suggested improvements. The parents of a learning disabled young man were neither asked to mediate nor to advise staff about appropriate language to use:

> I think, with hindsight, it might have been better if they had explained to us first...they actually direct everything towards the patient. So they don't actually direct anything towards the parents. The parent's more outside looking in because that's the way they run their treatment. (Father)

Of the four who banked, none remembered having a choice about *where* to produce the sample, for example at home, on the ward or at the sperm bank. Two had a choice about who to accompany them to the unit and were happy with their arrangements (both were accompanied by female family members). The other two were not offered a choice and were unhappy (one accompanied by a female family member and one by a male nurse). Lack of choice made it difficult for them to feel safe or supported in the way that worked best for them.

All four had views about the room itself. Professionals had wondered about whether to offer 'girlie' magazines. The two youngest at the time of banking both thought it was good to make them available, one did not and the fourth did not comment. One was concerned at the lack of privacy in the room whereas another (in a different centre) felt safe as it had an inside lock, window blinds and was soundproof. One had to use an unstable pot (which tipped over with the sample in it) as no alternative was offered. The need for a pre-agreed system for checking progress from time to time was also identified.

The pressure of decision-making and consenting

Although investigations ranged from a few weeks to eight months, few if any expected a cancer diagnosis and none knew beforehand that fertility may be affected by cancer treatment. However, the actual process of decision-making was experienced as relatively straightforward, even though pressured, and was seen as primarily about maintaining a route to fatherhood later in life.

Some remembered having to make the decision 'on the spot', with the longest time allowed being a week. As newly diagnosed patients, they were in shock and being given a lot of information in unfamiliar terms and language. Many found this affected their ability to handle the information and the decision. Three, including two who refused the offer, coped by putting the banking issues to the back of their mind:

> …you were getting told so much. You kind of had to put some things to the back of your mind and had to concentrate on some…and I think I kind of blanked it out… I wasn't thinking that far ahead. Just take one day at a time and then see what happens. (16 at diagnosis)

Parents felt their sons' understanding was limited (although they were not too concerned about this):

> …if I remember rightly he just got the piece of paper more or less just shoved in front of him… Well you don't get long to sign the paper do you… So I don't think he had time to think about it… He probably just signed and he didn't know what he was signing for at the time. (Mother)

Three young men felt that their physical state impinged:

> I didn't really have time cos as soon as they went out [of the room] it sort of went out of me head and I was busy being sick and that…the pain was terrible. So I don't think I was really all there… You just wait until they come back and then you just blurt out the answer you can be bothered to say. (16 at diagnosis)

All remembered that there was a consent form and knew where their copy was, but were less clear about its content:

> To be honest it went in one ear and out the other. It was just a load of jargon. I didn't understand it at all. All I understood was if I didn't sign this the sperm wouldn't be stored. (14 at diagnosis)

Only one had since had his fertility tested, revised his consent and felt clearer as a result.

Only one could remember signing the 'consent to disclosure' (Human Fertilisation and Embryology (Disclosure of Information) Act 1992) to allow information to go back to the paediatric oncology unit but all *assumed* that the paediatric oncology team were aware of the results.

The need for information

Respondents generally felt that they received good-enough, clearly presented information at the time of being invited to bank. All but one of the young men understood that they would have to masturbate; this was explained by paediatric oncology staff in language and at a level that they could comprehend, even though their ages at the time ranged from 14 to 17 and some had learning difficulties. However, few remembered being told beforehand how their sample would be stored if successful, or that a sample might not be suitable to freeze, or that they may fail to produce a sample at all. Several would have welcomed additional written and verbal information about what to do at the sperm bank to avoid confusion and distress:

> I was just walking around with it, walking up and down the corridor until I saw a doctor. It wasn't the one who actually referred me to the room, it was just any random doctor... It was a bit weird explaining to them what I had just been through and what do I do with it...and then they said just leave it in the room. So I had to go all the way back and put it in the same room... I didn't feel comfortable with it just lying around in a room that wasn't actually locked... I didn't know if it was safe or not because the doctor just told me leave it in the room then he walked off in a different direction. (16 at diagnosis)

Some parents also found the experience at the sperm bank difficult as they were unsure what to do and where to sit when their sons went through to be seen, and would have welcomed guidance.

Later issues such as how much had been stored, in what form and of what quality, actual effects of treatment on fertility, optimum times and methods for fertility testing, impact on sexual performance and relationships and the process and cost of using assisted conception treatments were also not covered very well, if at all, either at the time or later. Several would have welcomed additional written and verbal information, as would some parents who believed that they could help their sons more if they had better information and if they were involved differently by professionals.

The appropriate timing and frequency of making information available might be different for different people, as might the need for access to someone to talk to. Few knew whom they could approach for information after banking, either immediately or over time, and several said that they would welcome someone to talk to. Some parents thought they might want information earlier than their sons. It was of note that parents and sons both asked a number of factual questions about storage and treatment during the research interviews.

The significance of fertility preservation

The importance of being able to have children of one's own came through strongly and perhaps explains the young men's willingness to overcome significant barriers to banking. This was especially poignant for those who regretted not banking.

There were indications of shifting attitudes over time. One young man who did not bank said:

> While I was going through treatment I just totally forgot about it…
> I was coming back onto me radiotherapy…and I was thinking
> maybe if I had of done that, you know, maybe, I mean…it might not
> work later on in life. I might not be able to have kids because of it. So
> then I was thinking maybes I should have done it. (15 at diagnosis)

And a father said:

> We tend to think different about it now. At the time it was
> something, you just brush it away cos it's a decision he had to make.
> To us it was more important like whatever gonna get on we've got to
> get the cancer sorted out… But I mean in two years' time it will
> probably be a completely different conversation…but at that time
> and now…well it wasn't at the top of the pyramid.

It was a common experience that no one, including professionals, raised it again afterwards. One young man enquired about fertility testing shortly after treatment and was told to wait; it was never raised again. Two had talked about fertility in a more general way with their consultant, hoping it would prompt an offer of testing (it did not).

Many spoke of good, open relationships with professionals, citing consultants and social workers in particular as someone they potentially could talk to about fertility, but nevertheless found it too difficult to raise directly:

> It has just been good being able to talk about it really [in the research interview]. It's the first time I've been able to do it so it has been good, raising it… It's my first time [talking about it all]. (17 at diagnosis)

One mother described how she tried to 'manage' without using the professionals as she saw her needs as being less important than those of others:

> I didn't bother her [social worker] a lot but I kept thinking, you know, like she is seeing these people and sometimes their children's died and I'd still got […]. I cannot ring her up about that [fertility issues], that's silly. They say no, you're not bothering us, but I kept thinking I was bothering them about things.

One young man talked specifically about the impact of impaired fertility on his sexuality and another three wondered how it would affect romantic relationships:

> I haven't had a girlfriend since I was diagnosed so…I think if I did get a girlfriend having to tell them that I'm not going to be able to have kids or anything, that's going to be a bit of a shock to them isn't it so. Relationships, yeh, that's affected me getting in a relationship, getting the confidence to get a relationship anyway. (17 at diagnosis)

Several parents were aware of their sons' continuing distress at the impact on sexuality and fertility:

> …sometimes he would say well what happens if I can't have kids. You know everything's been ruined. Not just cos he got cancer just…you know, he likes kids; he keeps saying like probably nobody wants to marry us or, you know, he would never get a girlfriend because he couldn't have children and I said it is something you've just got to accept, if you can't have children, so… (Mother)

The importance of communication with professionals and others

Managing one's feelings through troubling times and the importance of communication with professionals was a major area for discussion. Many identified the manner and style of professionals that they either valued or found difficult.

The consensus was that the consultant was the most appropriate person to raise the issue of fertility preservation. Many had already started to form a trusting relationship even at this early stage and some positively recalled being encouraged to take more time to decide rather than going with their initial reaction.

Feeling embarrassed was a common and lasting reaction, but was eased where staff appeared comfortable, used humour, paid attention to privacy, showed kindness and compassion and were clear in their information sharing – and made more difficult where staff were clearly uncomfortable:

> ...she [nurse at the sperm bank] made us feel uncomfortable cos...she didn't seem very happy... Like you're not going to see them happy... She just like, this is going to happen...right here's the cup, go in there...just like that. Not like normal talking. (16 at diagnosis)

Phrasing of questions around consent was significant, for example when sperm bank staff asked what to do with banked sperm in the event of their death (a legal requirement in the UK). For two, this was made positive when it was pointed out that the question assumed they could live to age 55 and beyond; for a third, it was presented less sensitively and led to lasting distress:

> ...it could have been put more kindly I think...if you were to die... I had just found out I was diagnosed with it and the question comes up if you were to die... (16 at diagnosis)

Where information was put over well, the directness of the professional in giving information was appreciated, even though it could also be rather daunting:

> The doctors, they don't beat about the bush, they just like, right this is it. Then they just like say it. Then you have to look to think if that is what they've said or if you're just imagining it. (16 at diagnosis)

Some were able to manage this with great feeling:

When she [consultant] told me everything about it, it was quiet really, there was nobody else in the room and that's the way I preferred it as well…private, there was nobody else there…cos she actually drew the curtains and everything when she came in so it was very private, so that was good…yes that's what I preferred, anyway. I preferred being private without anybody listening in. (17 at diagnosis)

The consensus among both young men and parents was that the gender of the professional mattered less than the existence of a prior relationship or their general manner. Nevertheless, for some there was some uncertainty. Two young men said that they found it uncomfortable to talk with a woman about 'men's things' but one of these also struggled in his contact with the male nurse on the grounds that he did not know him.

One young man described his relief at talking to a fellow patient about their shared experiences in a late night conversation away at camp. Another felt similar relief when talking for the first time, more than two years later, to an adult who had banked. Just as poignantly, one had spoken with others on the ward at the time but, on realizing that they had all banked and he was not able to, did not feel able to discuss it again.

So what can be learnt from this?

In reproductive medicine, information about the immediate and longer-term experience of participating in medical advances often lags behind the technology. This study aimed to begin to address the gap in research knowledge about the experiences of young men under the age of majority and their parents when offered fertility preservation following cancer diagnosis.

As a pilot study designed to test the feasibility of interviewing those affected, the sample size was intended to be fairly small. Although take up of the study was high, the number of interviews conducted was actually lower than anticipated because of the high relapse rate within this patient population. The findings from the interviews alone should therefore be treated with caution; until more research is available we cannot know how typical are the experiences reported here. However, there were similarities with the findings from other parts of the study (interviews with professionals and national postal surveys of practice in paediatric oncology and assisted conception) that warrant attention and that suggest that face-to-face interviews on this sensitive topic have the potential to offer valuable additional information in helping to shape the future direction of services. Both young men and parents showed high levels of recall of their experiences and there were very few discrepancies between accounts.

Although there may well be room for debate about the level of understanding that is deemed sufficient to indicate competence in making this decision, and about the adequacy of the existing legal provision, *Gillick*[3] competence is currently a legal requirement for consent by minors in the UK, as are other aspects of the consent process. The lack of clarity among the young men and their parents about both consent to storage and consent to disclosure of information was perhaps due in part to the lack of clarity among some professionals (Crawshaw *et al.* 2003). When combined with the relative lack of written and verbal information, their understanding of the impact on their fertility and sexuality may be unnecessarily limited.

The need to pay more attention to increasing the choices available at the time of decision-making, albeit within unavoidable constraints, is important (Alderson 1994). Assumptions about the appropriateness of how to involve mothers and fathers, when to raise it, how and where the sample should be produced and who should accompany the young man to the sperm bank are all areas where there is room for improved professional attention to increasing choices, maximizing feelings of control (at a time when feelings of loss of control may be particularly high) and meeting individual need in patients and parents at this difficult time. This is not about proscribing what should happen, it is about using professional skill in communication together with provision of appropriate information to try and ensure that the process works well for the individual and parents concerned.

Offering greater choice does not mean abdicating responsibility for being proactive when appropriate. Respondents identified clear aspects of professional manner and communication that were valued highly, aided decision-making and made a difficult situation more manageable. These included directness and clarity in information giving, using warmth, and, on occasion, humour – and not being embarrassed.

Following the diagnosis period, there were indications that professionals either failed to raise the subject of fertility or any associated issues, including sexuality, directly or did so in a way that was too ambiguous or indirect for the young men to risk a response. In such a sensitive area, young men and their parents may need very explicit 'permission' to discuss any aspect of this whole area with the professional of their choice (which could potentially be anyone in the multi-disciplinary team) at a time of their choosing. For some, this may be quite early in the process and, for others, it may not be until they actively start to contemplate becoming sexually active or becoming parents. When teenagers are diagnosed with cancer, they are likely to miss significant amounts of schooling and may also find themselves dislocated from their previous peer and friendship groups. This may in turn reduce their access to information about sexual matters at an educative, social and emotional level. It is not clear whether parents and/or professionals can fill any of that gap but unless the need is acknowledged and attempts made by adults to build that bridge, then teenagers with cancer may be particularly disadvantaged.

Research elsewhere suggests that significant numbers of professionals do not feel competent in discussing sexual matters (Stead *et al.* 2001) and this is likely to be true in this context, especially with this age group. The professionals' interviews and the survey results showed a need for more staff training for working with this age group as well as a need for national written guidelines (see also Multi-disciplinary Working Group 2003).

Research in other areas of professional–patient/client communication has indicated that professionals sometimes fail to provide basic information (Eiser 1996; Weinman 1997). This was true at the time of sperm banking, including information about content (types of containers available, likelihood of producing a sample etc.) and process (where to sit, where to leave the sample etc.). These are complex areas to manage but need to be agreed in advance on an individual patient basis. Not only does this have the potential to reduce anxiety at the time but may also minimize the potential for lasting distress being generated.

The lack of age-appropriate written information on this subject is a significant difficulty for professionals, young men and parents alike. It is known that the amount of verbal information that is retained following professional encounters may be limited (Blacklay, Eiser and Ellis 1998; Bristol Royal Infirmary Inquiry 2001). Given the sensitive nature of fertility and sexuality, together with the fact that this subject is raised at or around diagnosis, the amount of information retained may be particularly low adding to the need to augment information through additional channels including written, audio-visual and web-based.

At a conference organized for more than 300 teenagers and young adults living with cancer in 2004, a colleague and I gave an early morning presentation on the final day and the room was packed. Throughout the entire conference, questions relating to fertility and sexuality came up time and time again. Living with the impact of this aspect of the cancer experience has received relatively scant attention to date and that needs to change. As one young woman who has been in remission for a number of years recently wrote:

> ...it's an incredible loss to feel like that's [fertility] been taken away from me...that's probably the hardest thing that I've had to deal with in my life, probably even more than the cancer... (Ivey 2004)

Notes

1 I would like to acknowledge the generosity of the teenagers and their parents in giving their time and sharing their experiences so openly in this study.

2 Devised by paediatric endocrinologist Dr Tanner, the Tanner Stages of development were developed by observing the pubic hair of males and females, the male genital area and the female breast. Stage 2 testes are reddened, thinner and larger (1.6–6 cc), for example.

3 *Gillick* competence is a term used in English medical law to describe the ruling made by the House of Lords in the case *Gillick* v. *West Norfolk and Wisbech Area Health Authority* 1985 3 ALL ER 402 (HL), relating to the rights of children under 16 to consent to medical treatment without their parents' knowledge.

10

Infertility

An Unspoken Presence in the Lives of Teens and Young Women with Turner Syndrome

Elizabeth Loughlin[1]

Introduction

> It would be fantastic if I could have children but that's an impractical
> want, some things are just meant to be. (Shauna, age 19)

Infertility is in the minds of girls and adolescents with Turner Syndrome (TS) but tends to be acknowledged in a few stock phrases. It is not until adult life that many of those living with TS find a language to describe this aspect of their genetic condition.

The chapter explores the unspoken presence of infertility in 12–16-year-olds, and then demonstrates, through case vignettes, the way that infertility began to take a central place for two young women with TS. It draws on my social work clinical experience with young people with TS, aged up to 16 years, referred from the endocrine out-patient clinic at the Royal Children's Hospital, Melbourne, Australia; a qualitative study of the experiences of three women with TS (Loughlin 1998; Loughlin and Werther 2000); and the perspectives of adult women members with TS from the Victorian Turner's Syndrome Association (VTSA).

What is Turner Syndrome?

Turner Syndrome is a common genetic condition found in approximately 1:2000 live female births. A syndrome means a collection of features and for those with TS this includes a combination of characteristic physical features and a complete or partial absence of the second sex (X) chromosome in some or all cells (Saenger *et al.* 2001). Described and named by Henry Turner (1938), nearly all those with the syndrome have short stature and insufficiently or non-functioning ovaries and thus face future infertility.

Their difference from peers is further complicated for some young people with TS who have additional features of chronic illness including serious heart problems, significant hearing loss, lymphoedema[2] and other symptoms. Although some girls with TS do not experience significant psycho-social issues, studies note a social immaturity in early adolescence and a tendency to draw back from social relationships (Swillen *et al.* 1993). Other girls can experience lowered self-image arising from the insensitive responses of their peers (Rickert *et al.* 1996). All have a childhood and adolescence in which regular medical review and treatment play a large part in their experience of growing up.

Hearing about the diagnosis

The following account is based on semi-structured discussions with the six individual hospital endocrinologists and one gynaecologist with whom I work. Girls are referred to the paediatric endocrinologist with symptoms such as puffy hands or feet in infancy, short stature in childhood, or delay in signs of puberty in teen years. The degree of focus on fertility in the initial appointments depends on the reason for the referral, the age at diagnosis, and whether or not there are other serious health features that need immediate treatment. In childhood, the medical focus is usually growth hormone treatment through daily injections to increase height, which is monitored by measurement of linear growth every three months. The mean untreated Caucasian adult height is 143–147 cm, approximately 4 ft 9 in (Elsheikh *et al.* 2002). With treatment many girls grow to a height in the low normal range. From around the age of puberty, the medical focus turns to the use of sex hormone replacement therapy (HRT) to induce secondary sex characteristics including breast development, and regular checks continue.

Learning about infertility

In our hospital, the diagnosis of Turner Syndrome is told to the girl and her parents together. Commonly, parents and their daughters have not heard of the syndrome nor know that it affects ovarian function. One study found that almost all parents (90%) find it difficult to cope with their daughter's infertility (Slijper *et al.* 1998). Published family stories and anecdotes show that parents are devastated by the information that normal ovaries are not present and that their daughter is unlikely to have her own child (Karamesinis 2003; Turner Syndrome Support Society, UK 2002).

In my practice experience with families, the mother is shocked and often cries in the clinic consults. She thinks of the grandchildren she and her husband will never have. She mourns for her daughter's future loss often well ahead of the daughter's own sense of loss. The father is upset but may focus on his daughter's external appearance 'as long as she is happy and looks OK', although he can grieve silently. Girls feel for their mother's distress and may not wish to distress them further with questions about their own confusion.

At the age of puberty or when HRT is introduced, the doctor explains or re-explains to the girl that the ovaries will be unable to produce egg follicles, and that having babies 'in the usual way' is not possible. At the same time the doctor offers the girl and her parents encouraging information about alternative routes to forming a family, for example through *in vitro* fertilization (IVF) using egg donation or through adoption. One of my medical colleagues emphasizes to her adolescent patients the similarities they have with other young women – namely the ability to carry a pregnancy, give birth and breast feed. She may talk over the pros and cons of using a known or an unknown egg donor even at this early stage, but notes that her patients do not necessarily ask for further details until much later.

For some girls and parents, learning about the fertility status is more hopeful; 2–5 per cent of girls will have spontaneous menses and may have the potential to achieve pregnancy without medical intervention (Saenger *et al.* 2001). For some others, infertility is more final; in approximately 6 per cent of girls one of the sex chromosome contains Y material (Elsheikh *et al.* 2002) and both gonads develop as rudimentary testes rather than ovaries, and are surgically removed due to the risk of malignancy.

At approximately age 16–18 years, most endocrinologists refer their patients to our hospital gynaecology clinic – which is staffed entirely by women – for more detailed discussion of fertility status, IVF and continuing review of health and older adolescent concerns. In particular the gynaecologist will gently explore issues over the next few years that may arise around relationships, sexuality and infertility. The gynaecology clinic consults with young women up to 24 years, thus offering a supportive transitional time before referral to the adult specialist or adult hospital clinic.

Experiencing infertility

There are few studies in the extensive professional literature on TS that ask women with TS about their thoughts on the infertility, or their experiences of adoption or IVF. Sylven *et al.* (1993) found in semi-structured interviews with 22 women that half (11) said infertility was the most difficult part of having TS. In their study of 63 women, Wide Boman *et al.* (2000) reported that out of 55 (87%) who remembered their reaction to the diagnosis of TS, 49 (78%) reported negative consequences of having TS, with infertility as one of the consequences most often mentioned. Tang (1989), in a study of 86 Chinese women, found that for 51 per cent (44) the stigma of infertility appeared a cultural barrier to marriage or relationships. Kagan-Kreiger (1999), in her qualitative study of eight women with TS aged 23–44 years, found that most of them needed to rethink or revisit their feelings about their infertility, sometimes with the help of therapy, in order to ameliorate its impact on their relationships and self-image and to come to terms with themselves as women. In my own qualitative phenomenological study of three women with TS (Loughlin 1998) one woman aged 47 felt that the lack of clarity about her infertility, along with misunderstanding of her diagnosis, was detrimental to her sexuality and marriage; another woman, aged 26, experienced infertility as a major issue that affected her adjustment to TS; and for the third woman, aged 19, infertility had a daily presence in her mind.

Orten and Orten (1994) reported on the direct effect of fertility status on adult women with TS and their relationships. They found that a persistent concern of women in the TS support group was about how to tell a prospective male partner about their infertility. A recurrent theme with adult women from the TS support group in Melbourne was continuing regret that they could not meet with what they felt was society's expectation that women should become mothers (Loughlin 1993).

No published studies of adolescent attitude to loss of fertility through TS were found.

Involving the social worker

In our hospital, the endocrinologists refer girls with TS and their parents to me as the social worker on the endocrine team for counselling at the time of diagnosis, or at any time when personal or social issues arise. In addition to individual counselling, I offer peer group counselling experiences to teens with TS to address their concern about their physical differences from others and any teasing that they may be experiencing in school. As a trained dance and creative arts therapist, I use creative interventions additional to verbal interventions as a way to access the feelings and thoughts that may be too hard to express in words.

I often find that, in childhood, the girl's preoccupation is with growth. Kelly (all names have been changed) was diagnosed at nine years:

> I just hoped I didn't have to have injections, and the next appointment the doctor said I did!

For girls with TS, infertility recedes into the background but even so is still remembered. Natalie, now 18 and looking back, told me:

> I knew when I was about seven I think. Mum told me. Time to sink in, when it didn't matter as much.

Girls diagnosed in their early to mid-teen years, on the other hand, have to take in the doctors' information about growth, puberty development and infertility at the same time. Through the teen group counselling programme, several of the girls were able to tell me more about their reactions to finding out about TS at this time of life. Nola learned about her diagnosis at 15 years and told me that it made her scared. Linette learned at 13 when she came to hospital for another investigation; she said it made her feel so mixed up she did not know how to feel. Geraldine learned at 14 years; she said she was shocked but relieved when the doctor explained it all. Marie knew at 11 and was also relieved to find out why she was short, but said it really annoyed her. Yet they often find it hard to expand further on how they feel. They sometimes find it easier to refer to their mother's response to their future infertility:

> My mother cried so much at the doctor's and when she came home too.

> My mother said I coped better than her. She thought it was her fault.

For young women of 16 years and over who have been referred later to the specialist, the experience of hearing that they have a syndrome and are unlikely to conceive can be overwhelming. One young woman of 16 told me that she felt her life had been a lie that hid the truth of who she really was. Following diagnosis, she felt that she was a completely different person from the one she had always been. Several others have spoken in a similar way of reacting with shock and anger, becoming reluctant to talk, withdrawing into themselves and preferring to cope on their own.

The impact of infertility

So what can social work interventions and research tell us about the impact of infertility? The following section examines data collected and analysed from my clinical social work practice and research to begin to explore the place of fertility and its impact on teens and young women with TS.

This section is divided developmentally into three parts:

1. Preoccupations of girls 12–16 years attending the group counselling programmes.

2. The views of young women late adolescence to mid-twenties.

3. The perspective from adult women mid-thirties to sixties.

The preoccupations of girls 12–16 years attending the group counselling programmes

The teen group programme is an eight to ten-hour programme held over three to five consecutive weeks each year. The average attendance is seven girls who for the most part are referred from the hospital clinic and have attended prior individual counselling with me. The following data are drawn from four such group programmes, which included 21 girls, six of whom attended a second group programme another year.

The aims of the programme are to improve self-esteem; to enable participants to move out into the world with confidence; to provide the space to talk over the ups and downs of having TS; and to enjoy themselves with others.

The clinical approach is psychotherapeutic counselling, using both verbal and non-verbal interventions within a framework of the 'lived' experiencing body in chronic illness (Leder 1992). I developed the creative intervention demonstrated below as an adjunct to hospital social work verbal counselling. In this instance the group participants were invited to make a floor design from a large variety of objects about an open-ended topic, for example 'About me' or 'My progress'. A process of phenomenological verbal questioning (Betensky 1987) expands the meaning of the topic: *look at your design, describe what you 'see'; what stands out most; what parts are connected to each other; what title would you give your work?* This particular creative exercise can also be a marker for the young person and the social worker to note the development of themes over time.

In the discussion and conversations about themselves, infertility was rarely brought up verbally, but some girls expressed it visually. The following illustrated designs and accompanying descriptive words are from the second group programme.

Infertility: an unspoken presence

In the creative floor design 'About me' two out of six girls referred to their fertility status. In session one Katherine (13) carefully selected scarves and objects to make her design. Then, in response to my questions, she verbally described her work referring in the main to her infertility and its impact.

> The yellow ribbon is the body. Inside the ribbon the solid objects are emotions. The things under the scarves are the organs [ovaries] that don't work.

She called her work *My secret inner emotions* (see Figure 10.1).

In the second session, Katherine looked at a photo of her creative design from the previous week and saw her creation in a wider positive perspective.

> I notice that the veils and the golden parts stand out more – I see the blood that keeps me alive.

Linette (14) came from a large family and in fact had spontaneous menses, which theoretically indicated the potential for fertility. This preoccupied her and her mother. In session one Linette created a design about having a child. She selected soft materials to make a small and large facial outline, and said:

> My design has two smiling faces.

In the second session she continued her description of this design:

> The child looks brighter, like a clown, really happy. The mother is older and more sophisticated and mature.

In the fifth and final session, Linette's new design repeated the theme of the child, but in a more abstract way (see Figure 10.2):

> I've always wanted twins and the two [artificial] apples are the two babies.

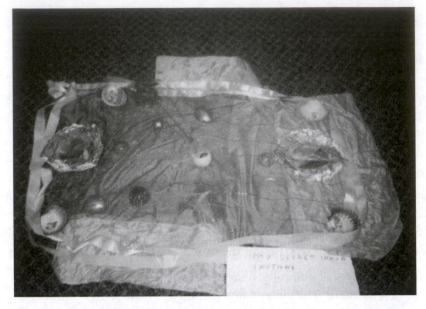

Figure 10.1 Katherine – My secret inner emotions

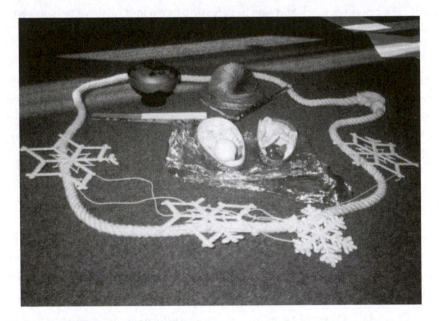

Figure 10.2 Linette – The twins

For Katherine and Linette, their design and description was a means to express something of their sadness and hope, respectively, about their future.

No language to ask questions about fertility

In the first group programme a young married woman of 21 with TS came and spoke to the participants about her own adolescence and young adult-hood and how she worked through her issues. The group participants asked her questions about how it felt for her to be short and what it was like to be different. However, when the young woman moved on to describe her future plans for IVF this usually talkative group of teens, who had found it hard to form a prepared question on this topic, also found it hard to ask her a question spontaneously during the discussion time. When she described how she would ask her sister for an egg, one participant said softly:

It's the same genes.

In the fourth group programme, fertility was introduced as a specific discussion topic. Deirdre (16) put the topic aside:

I don't think about the future, like fertility, too much.

And Yvonne (14) said:

It doesn't mean a lot to me yet.

Kerrie (13) had thought of possible solutions when she summed up her thoughts thus:

When I was ten, my friend and I decided she would have a baby for me.

In these sessions, there was more interest in discussing current concerns; for example, how they were keeping up with other girls at school or whether someone at school was being nasty to them in some way.

The loss of fertility may be too hard to imagine or to speak about as it is a loss that belongs to future experience. Furthermore, the teens in the group programmes seemed more preoccupied with the 'observable' body – what they saw as their physical difference from their peers (Loughlin 2000).

Physical difference

Kelly from the same group programme as Katherine and Linette made a cre-ative design about herself that seemed to reflect her perception that she sometimes felt different from others. In session one she selected and arranged a purple ribbon and other objects to make her design. She finally placed a small woollen lamb in the centre and covered it with a chiffon see-through scarf. She described her design:

> The lamb underneath the scarf is like me – I'm the odd one out.

She gave her design the title *This is me?* (see Figure 10.3).

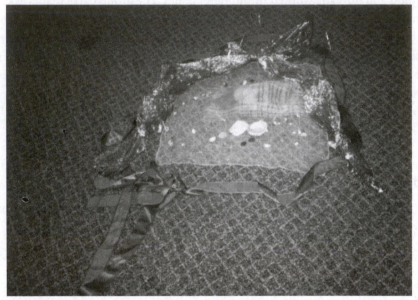

Figure 10.3 Kelly – This is me?

Her floor design in the fifth and final session was similar in style. Kelly said her design was about the:

> …pretty things which are separated from those that are not so pretty.

She continued looking at her design but chose to say no more about its meaning. She titled her design: *Symbols* (see Figure 10.4). Four years later her creative designs still resonated for her. She said:

> I have those photos at home. I look at them sometimes. I really said a lot then, didn't I? (Clinical notes)

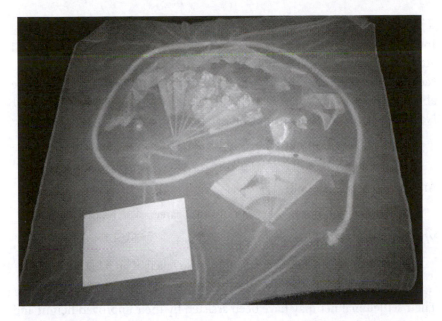

Figure 10.4 Kelly – Symbols

At the beginning of the third group programme the teenagers brought up their embarrassment and angst at their physical difficulties:

> People stare at my hands; they are puffy. The other girls have pretty fingers. (Tammy referring to her lymphoedema)

> My wrists don't work for ballgames – I'm not an asset in the group. (Wendy's skeletal problems)

> I can't roll in the gym. (Simone, difficulty in coordination)

> People say I can't run properly. (Tilly is overweight)

Nancy summed up the way she felt different from her peers in what could be a sense of shame:

> The spotlight is on you, I want to hide.

These physical preoccupations, together with earlier teasing about their short stature, contribute to confusion and uncertainty about their body over and above the usual adolescent concerns. These preoccupations need to be named and addressed in various mediums before infertility, as a significant part of the social and emotional body, can begin to find a verbal expression.

The views of young women late adolescence to mid-twenties

In follow-up conversations with a number of young women who had attended the group programme several years before, the young women seemed more comfortable with their syndrome and spoke with an ease about the place of infertility in their minds, although still in a summary way. Natalie (18) said about her infertility status:

> I'm pretty well getting my head around it – it's not a problem at the moment.

Another, Teresa (18), said:

> I really believe I have other options of a career.

While a third, Kelly (19), said:

> Knowing my prospects so early it's not so much of an issue, but it's in the back of my mind, with the alternatives. (Clinical notes)

Their settled manner may have been assisted by their improved height and also the well-being that is said to accompany growth hormone, together with the confidence engendered by the availability of IVF, and the opportunities for frank peer discussion through the clinical group programme.

However, few young women in my counselling group programmes appear to actively seek website information on fertility (www.mivf.com.au) and few in this age group attend the VTSA formal seminars on fertility and other related topics.

Is the issue of fertility still 'on hold' for them? Or does infertility plus a chronic health condition plus a tendency to socially 'draw back' mean there are too many layers to unravel in order to think about the impact of infertility on their future or to communicate their concerns to health advisors and friends?

Qualitative research is one way to ascertain the meaning of living with the many layered experiences of a chronic illness (Leder 1992). In my qualitative research project (Loughlin 1998) issues of infertility emerged as an important part of the experiencing of TS and here I present vignettes of the two younger women, Shauna (19) and Kate (26), to illustrate. This study also used creative interventions – movement and drawing – as a bridge to experiences. Data consisted of the participants' verbal descriptions of their movement patterns, drawings and accompanying thoughts and feelings. The descriptions were transcribed to create a verbal text that was analysed with systematic phenomenological procedures (Giorgi 1989; Moustakas

1994) to find the meanings in the individuals' life experiences. The two following vignettes are drawn from the study's synthesized summary descriptions and quotes from the transcripts. They offer more detail than clinical anecdote of the place of infertility in the lives of two young women with TS.

Vignette 1: Shauna, age 19

Shauna is a confident university student, engaged to be married. Diagnosed at birth, she learned about TS early on:

> I can't separate 'Shauna' from Turner Syndrome as I've known Turner's all my life.

In her early childhood she was cared for by others when her mother was often hospitalized with illness. The family moved around a lot and she frequently changed schools. She had repeated hospital stays for facial surgery and other surgery connected with her condition. Shauna always felt supported by her female endocrinologist and other doctors; she gained strength from her parents' acceptance of her condition and their desire to help *her* to accept her condition. On the subject of fertility, she feels that:

> Some people with TS blow fertility out of proportion. We already know, so we have a chance to come to terms with it. We have to get on with it.

Nevertheless her infertility has a distinct presence in her life:

> It was hard for my parents and me when I had my ovaries removed and they had to tell me that I couldn't have children... I love playing with children and it would be fantastic if I could have children but that's an impractical want...some things are just meant to be... I am very fortunate that I've got nieces and nephews to play with and I love them as if they were my own. (Transcript Shauna, data session two, Loughlin 1998)

Nevertheless, the sadness of infertility and the efforts to be positive influence her life as a young woman:

> I am not just the energetic happy-go-lucky person. I feel I'm treading on a tightrope.

In the next vignette Kate, 26, has a different experience of both her syndrome and the impact of infertility on her life.

Vignette 2: Kate, age 26

Kate is a well-educated, articulate young woman with a smart appearance that covers her struggle to control a body that she distrusts and that she feels lets her down. At times she is physically unwell. Kate was diagnosed at age seven and her parents told her 'everything' at age ten. She felt her experience of TS was negatively influenced by having ongoing medical reviews and by the constant pressure to 'measure up' to a height increase that her doctor and parents wanted. At school there were always reminders of her different height and body shape. She described the contradiction between being short and infertile yet attaining physical development and periods through female hormone medication, and also the contradiction between her chronological age and her younger physical appearance. Contradictions extended to social behaviour:

> There's a struggle between how I am naturally, what I want to be and what I think society expects from someone of my physique.

As a young woman she placed infertility, along with the body and sexuality, in a metaphorical 'box' in her mind in order to control and contain her feelings about her physical self. Kate did not find the new developments of IVF encouraging and expressed her viewpoint strongly:

> I had fertility taken away from me. If the IVF does not work, it will be taken away from me all over again.

Kate thought she could not identify with infertility as a separate issue:

> The bottom line is Turner's, its effects and its consequences – it's not the shortness per se, it's not the infertility per se, it's the whole package.

For Shauna, the early emotional disruptions in childhood and issues associated with repeated surgery, alongside support from her family and hospital doctor, seem to have given her a determination to adapt to the condition, to think about infertility and to move forward. Shauna was also young enough to have growth hormone treatment and to be part of a somewhat more optimistic milieu of assisted reproduction that implies more choice for adult women with TS. For Kate, just a few years older, growth hormone had not been available. As Kate did not attend the hospital clinic she did not have the early hospital counselling opportunity to talk about the lack of control over the body that she experienced in her childhood and adolescent medical reviews, or even to talk over teasing and being short. Sinason (1992) writes about the alienation of some people from their bodies when there is a trauma to the body of a physical or social kind. She postulates that after the primary trauma, there can be a secondary trauma, which may have been present for Kate in her mid-twenties as a result of not speaking about or understanding the original insult to her body.

The perspective from adult women mid-thirties to sixties

To explore the place of fertility from a longer perspective, I invited adults with TS from the VTSA, through their newsletter, to a semi-structured group discussion on the topic of fertility (Loughlin 2004). Five women accepted. They ranged in age from mid-thirties to early sixties; two were married with adopted children, one was married with no plans for children, a fourth was unmarried, and a fifth was engaged to be married and interested in IVF.

Fertility began to matter to the women in their late teens and early twenties although three had learned about it in their early teens. Of these, one woman said it mattered to her after the end of her first marriage at 24; two others said it mattered to them at 17 and 19 years. The other two women had only learned later about their syndrome (at 16 and 20 respectively) and infertility mattered to them straight away. But even then, as one woman said:

> It was not on my mind a terrible lot, I thought I'd cross that bridge when I come to it – it was a mighty bridge.

The five women said, looking back, infertility impacted on their self-worth, self-esteem or on making new relationships. One woman referred to TS impacting on sexuality:

> It's more unsureness about the missing X chromosome. Am I a full woman? Can I have a full sexual relationship?

Four particularly described the fear as a young woman of telling a future boyfriend, as Orten and Orten (1994) had found in their study:

> How will he take me out (4 ft 8 in) when there are girls who are 6 ft, blonde and gorgeous?

And:

> Once you have a serious relationship, it hits home. The rubber hits the bitumen.

And also:

> Sometimes one thinks I'm not even going to bother approaching that person.

These words link fertility with sexuality and also seem to suggest that these women saw themselves, perhaps earlier, as diminished in some way by the fact of their syndrome-induced infertility.

Other people were cited as helpful in adjusting to their infertility:

> My aunt.

> Having a baby sister.

> Nieces and nephews. (Echoing Shauna's reliance on relationships with her very young relatives)

> Meeting someone really disabled.

> Joining the Association and talking to others.

> Friends and new friends.

The women also said they had relied on themselves and their own strengths:

> Telling myself: 'Don't let it overtake your life, there are other things to do.'

And:

> It's a private matter, ultimately you have to work through it and deal with it in your own way.

Earlier medical advisors were remembered largely as 'not helpful', although all the women were pleased with their current gynaecologists. They said that when they were younger, there was a stigma about counselling. Adoption had been suggested as an alternative route to motherhood for the married older women (when they were younger), and now IVF for the two women in their thirties. One woman referred to a child-free life as an alternative:

> I've travelled my own road... I have been a free agent to go anywhere.

Fostering and inter-country adoption were not mentioned in this discussion and neither were the considerable risks in pregnancy for those with serious heart problems, although they are thoroughly discussed in the scientific literature.

Even though age and experience seemed to ameliorate the effect of infertility, the women's statements suggested a depth of feeling that was still present from an earlier age. On a one to ten scale of difficulty, with ten the most difficult, fertility was an issue for all five women when they were in the 18–20 age group. Now in the present, one woman in her thirties rated it at four and the second woman in her thirties rated it at nine. The three women 40+ rated infertility at six to eight in their thirties but at one in their forties. This clearly indicates the significant place (as with other women) of fertility difficulties in the child-bearing years of women with TS. One woman's response resonated with all the other women:

> Infertility is one of the cruellest things of Turner Syndrome, the choice was taken from me.

Comment

Infertility is an unspoken shadow that is always present for girls and adolescents with TS from the time of diagnosis at whatever age. The impact of infertility can be masked by the teens' preoccupation with their physical differences from their peers, and also for some by the need to focus on the chronic illness features of their condition. The difficulty for the young person with TS is finding a language to name and express feelings about infertility. By a woman's mid-thirties, when wisdom from life-experience permits more verbal exploration, it may be too late for her to think about assisted reproduction.

Even when fertility is possible through reproductive technology, thoughts may still be hard to form. One young mother with TS (28) described her IVF experience as:

> A huge sense of overwhelming me. I was changing a whole life of thinking I could not have kids – that was the real struggle. The procedures were easy.

A further dilemma is the need for young women to move on from the helpful and optimistic information, received in the paediatric setting about alternative ways to become a mother, in order to face the pain and disappointment that unsuccessful plans for adoption or IVF in adult life may bring. Given that some adolescents and young women with TS have a tendency to 'draw back' from social encounters including with their professional helpers, it is important that both verbal and more innovative ways are available for them to express the meanings of infertility and acknowledge their loss. Furthermore it is important that young women feel free to explore fertility as a metaphor for the creation of new things or new relationships in their life, especially if they choose not to or cannot become a mother.

Notes

1 Thank you to the teen girls who gave permission to reproduce their artwork, to the women who were subjects for my research project, to the VTSA and their members for their interest and willingness to share their memories, and to the RCH endocrinologists and gynaecologist for their participation in the doctor questionnaire.

2 Where excess fluid collects in the tissue and causes swelling.

11

Sexual and Reproductive Health in Young People with Cystic Fibrosis
Hard to Talk About but too Important to Ignore

Bridget Farrant and Susan Sawyer

Introduction

> My mother told me I couldn't have kids but at the time I wasn't sure what she meant, whether it was having kids or having sex. (Older adolescent male with cystic fibrosis)

Cystic fibrosis (CF) is a severe, chronic, life-limiting, multi-organ genetic disorder that exacts a heavy toll on adolescents due to the time-consuming nature of daily treatments. In the 1960s, when the median survival of people born with CF was 12 years (Phelan, Allen and Barnes 1979), there was little focus on sexual and reproductive health complications. However, the past few decades of improved medical care now result in an expectation of survival through adolescence into adult life. Indeed, the median survival is over 30 years in most specialized CF clinics (Dodge *et al.* 1997). Increasing survival has changed the relative importance and relevance of many of the health effects of CF, especially in relationship to sexual and reproductive health. While there have been significant advances in understanding and management of various sexual and reproductive health complications in young people with CF, there is still much scope for improvement in health care services to ensure that young people and their families are sensitively informed about these issues in a developmentally appropriate and timely manner.

CF is inherited as an autosomal recessive condition[1] that affects approximately 1:2500 Caucasian live births, with lower rates in other ethnic groups (e.g. 1:15,000 Africans and 1:30,000 Asians). Approximately 1:25 fit and healthy people are asymptomatic carriers for the disorder (Dodge *et al.* 1997). It is caused by mutations in the CF transmembrane regulator gene, which encodes the CFTR protein that is responsible for ion and water transport across cells in different glands and organ systems in the body. Absence of the CFTR protein results in various cellular abnormalities that, over time, result in organ damage and loss of function.

The primary impact of CF is on the respiratory system where the production of abnormal mucus predisposes to persistent lower respiratory tract infection, bronchiectasis[2] and obstructive airways disease, with progressive loss of respiratory function over time. Regular physiotherapy and antibiotics ameliorate but do not cure progressive respiratory disease. Where available, lung transplantation can prolong life in those with end stage disease, but respiratory failure remains the leading cause of death. Another major impact of CF is on the gastrointestinal system. In over 90 per cent of people with CF, malabsorption and malnutrition result from pancreatic enzyme deficiency. Supplementation with pancreatic enzymes normalizes the absorptive defect, although a high energy diet is still required. There are many other associations and complications of CF as outlined in Table 11.1.

Young people with CF face the same range of sexual and reproductive health issues as people without CF. They generally commence sexual activity at the same median age as healthy young people (Sawyer, Phelan and Bowes 1995). However, there are specific sexual and reproductive complications of CF that are an additional challenge for adolescents, as outlined in Figure 11.1. Some of these, such as pubertal delay, are common to both males and females; others are gender-specific, such as infertility in males and urinary incontinence in females. The sexual and reproductive health complications of CF are also a mix of congenital co-morbidities such as male infertility, and acquired complications such as yeast infections in females.

The focus of this chapter is on the issue of (in)fertility and reproduction for young people with CF.

Table 11.1 Multi-system manifestations of CF

Respiratory	Bronchiectasis (progressive loss of respiratory function, haemoptysis,[a] pneumothorax,[b] respiratory failure)
	Allergic bronchopulmonary aspergillosis[c]
	Pneumothorax
	Nasal polyps
	Chronic sinusitis
Gastrointestinal	Pancreatic insufficiency
	Diabetes mellitus
	Distal Intestinal Obstruction Syndrome[d]
	Rectal prolapse
	Recurrent pancreatitis
	Liver disease (focal biliary cirrhosis,[e] fatty infiltration, oesophageal varices,[f] hypersplenism[g])
	Gastroesophageal reflux[h]
Bones and joints	Clubbing
	Arthritis
	Osteoporosis
Sweat glands	Salt loss syndrome
Genitourinary	See Figure 11.1

Notes

a The spitting of blood from the lungs or bronchial tubes as a result of pulmonary or bronchial haemorrhage.

b Abnormal collection of air outside the lining of the lung and chest wall.

c An allergic reaction to a fungus called aspergillus, which causes inflammation of the airways and air sacs.

d Obstruction of the intestine due to overly thick meconium, the dark sticky stuff normally present at birth. Previously called meconium ileus.

e Slow destruction of the bile ducts within the liver.

f Swollen veins in the walls of the gullet. Fragile and tend to bleed easily.

g Enlarged spleen and a decrease in one or more type of blood cells.

h Gastric juice backs up into the oesophagus.

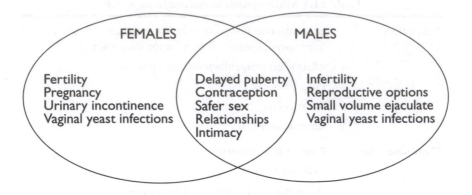

FEMALES

Fertility
Pregnancy
Urinary incontinence
Vaginal yeast infections

Delayed puberty
Contraception
Safer sex
Relationships
Intimacy

MALES

Infertility
Reproductive options
Small volume ejaculate
Vaginal yeast infections

Figure 11.1 Sexual and reproductive health effects of CF

Psycho-social development in young people with CF

Growing up with a chronic illness such as CF has both a physical and emotional toll on young people's psycho-social development. The growth and pubertal delay common in CF has been shown to have a negative effect on young people's self-esteem and body image and other people's perception of their age and development (Sawyer *et al.* 1995). This is further complicated by the other obvious physical markers of CF, such as surgical scars, the visibility of permanent intravenous access ports and body habitus such as a barrel-shaped chest. These can all interfere with young people's development of peer and romantic relationships, and perception of physical attractiveness and self-worth (Sawyer 2000; Sawyer *et al.* 1995). The urinary incontinence experienced by many women with CF has also been shown to affect young women's social life and intimate relationships negatively (Nixon *et al.* 2003). Emotionally, growing up with a life-limiting condition has been shown to influence some young people into more risk-taking activities (e.g. early and unprotected sexual activity), while for others it may lead to lack of emotional development, dependence on caregivers and poor maturity of relationship with peers or intimate relationships (Sawyer 2000; Surís, Michaud and Viner 2004). While some studies have found that, overall, groups of young people with CF have the same average age of onset of sexual activity, same level of sexual activity and the same rates of marriage/de facto relationships as otherwise healthy peers (Sawyer,

Phelan and Bowes 1995; Sawyer *et al.* 1995), it is worth noting that other studies have found that young people with CF reported an avoidance of close relationships in adolescence and a delay in intimacy due to concern about their partner's reaction to their illness (Johannessen *et al.* 1998). Reassuringly, Johannessen *et al.* (1998) also report that the majority of these young people were able to establish intimate relationships as adults.

Male infertility

Approximately 98 per cent of males with CF are infertile. The genetic abnormality that results in CF is associated with aberrant embryological development of the reproductive portion of the mesonephric (wolffian) duct. At birth, this results in variable absence of the vas deferens, seminal vesicle, ejaculatory duct and body and tail of the epididymis[3] (see Figure 11.2). While active spermatogenesis occurs in the testis, sperm are unable to be transported from the testis due to congenital absence of the vas deferens (Kaplan *et al.* 1968; McCallum *et al.* 2000). Neither sex hormone production nor sexual function are affected.

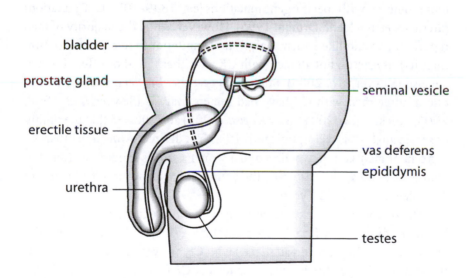

Figure 11.2 Male genitourinary anatomy in CF

As a result of this transport defect, men with CF were previously unable to have children. Recent developments in reproductive technology now enable infertile men with CF to achieve biological paternity through aspiration of sperm from the epididymis (microsurgical epididymal sperm aspiration or MESA) or from the testis itself (testicular sperm aspiration or TESA) in association with intracytoplasmic sperm injection (ICSI) (see Chapter 6). The use of these techniques in couples where the male has CF has resulted in pregnancy rates of 30–35 per cent per cycle, with 62.5 per cent of couples achieving pregnancy following the treatment programme (McCallum *et al.* 2000; Rosenlund *et al.* 1997). These are expensive technologies that are only available in specialized assisted reproduction centres (and at variable expense to the affected couple). In a recent survey of males with CF in Australia, nearly 20 per cent of adult men had children (Sawyer *et al.* 2005). Six had fathered children using assisted reproductive techniques (MESA), nine had used donor insemination and one had stepchildren. Another man was presumed to be fertile having fathered a child without technological assistance.

Investigation of male fertility status using semen analysis is important, as a minority of men with CF (some few per cent only) will be fertile. This is more common with specific gene mutations (e.g. 3849-10kb C-T mutation) (Stern, Doershuck and Drumm 1995). However, while the majority of men report they would like semen analysis to be undertaken in order to confirm their fertility status, not all men with CF are either tested or offered semen analysis (Sawyer *et al.* 2005). Studies suggest that between one in two and one in three men with CF have had semen analysis (Sawyer *et al.* 1998, 2005; Thickett *et al.* 2001). Sawyer *et al.* (2005) also showed that the timing of semen analysis is still significantly later than desired: while more than 95 per cent of men said they believed that semen analysis should be offered to men before the age of 20 years, the youngest age of testing in this recent Australian study was 24 years.

The first studies to explore any aspect of the sexual and reproductive health needs of men with CF date from the late 1980s. These early studies showed that adolescent and adult men with CF had very poor knowledge of the sexual and reproductive complications of CF (Hames, Beesley and Nelson 1991; Nolan *et al.* 1986). Of note, Hames *et al.* (1991) found that the majority of both males and their parents were unaware that men with CF were infertile. More recent studies from the last decade in Boston, USA (Sawyer *et al.* 1998), Birmingham, England (Thickett *et al.* 2001), Scotland

(Fair, Griffiths and Osman 2000) and Australia (Sawyer *et al.* 2005) have shown increasing awareness of infertility in men with CF: the majority of contemporary men with CF know that their fertility is likely to be affected by the disorder, and know why this is so. These studies also identify that between 68 and 84 per cent of men with CF want children in the future. The desire for more information on sexual and reproductive health is a consistent theme across studies (Fair *et al.* 2000; Sawyer *et al.* 2005; Thickett *et al.* 2001). However, despite the improved survival of CF over the past few decades, few studies have directly assessed the impact of future infertility on teenagers with CF. Apart from a qualitative US study (Sawyer *et al.* 1998) that included ten adolescent males (of whom five were not aware of male infertility), our knowledge of the impact of infertility in adolescence has been obtained from the (retrospective) reflections of adult men with CF. This qualitative study informed the development of a quantitative survey of adult men with CF in Australia (Sawyer *et al.* 2005). Both studies suggest that knowledge of infertility in adolescence is less overwhelming than might be thought. For example, 90 per cent of men reported not being distressed when they first heard about infertility during adolescence (Sawyer *et al.* 1998). Typical comments were:

> There was no real effect at the time. I just took it as part of CF.
> (29-year-old who first heard about likely infertility when aged 12)

And:

> I didn't really think about it much. At the time I wasn't upset.
> (27-year-old who first heard when 15)

However, 10 per cent described a significant impact upon hearing of male infertility in adolescence. For example, one said:

> It took me by surprise, I was shocked. (25-year-old who was first told when he was 12)

The impact of infertility appears to become more significant as adolescents and young adults mature and form more intimate and committed relationships where there is an expectation of fertility (Sawyer *et al.* 1998, 2005). Typical comments were:

> At first it went in one ear and out the other, but then I thought about it. (20-year-old)

And:

> At the moment it's not a concern. It's like it hasn't really hit me yet.
> Later, it could be devastating. (19-year-old)

Infertility was reported as an insignificant aspect of CF by only 10 per cent of adult men. For example, one commented:

> I've been busy with living, which is more important than having kids. (38-year-old) (Sawyer *et al.* 1998)

Female reproduction

In contrast to men with CF, adolescent and adult women have anatomically normal reproductive tracts. While fertility may be reduced due to thickened cervical mucous and the potential anovulatory effects of severe respiratory disease and malnutrition, fertility should be assumed to be normal until proven otherwise (Sawyer 2000). Exact fertility rates are unknown, as many women with CF choose not to become pregnant, citing concerns about the impact of pregnancy, the time and energy required to care for a young child on their health and concern that the child may have CF (Odegaard *et al.* 2002; Sawyer, Phelan and Bowes 1995). Early reports of fertility rates as little as 20 per cent normal (Kopito, Kosasky and Shwachman 1973) are most unlikely, as recent studies have shown that up to three-quarters of women who tried to become pregnant were successful (Odegaard *et al.* 2002; Sawyer, Phelan and Bowes 1995). Reports of unplanned pregnancy (Hull and Kass 2000; Kotloff, FitzSimmons and Fiel 1992; Sawyer, Phelan and Bowes 1995) further reinforce that young women should assume their fertility is normal. This has obvious repercussions for contraception, especially for teenage girls. In the past, mistaken beliefs of female infertility placed adolescent and adult women at risk of unplanned pregnancy because of the failure to use appropriate contraception (Sawyer, Phelan and Bowes 1995). Continuing high rates of termination of pregnancy in women with mild as well as severe lung disease suggests that lack of attention to effective contraception continues to be a problem (Goss *et al.* 2003).

The more contentious issue has been the safety of pregnancy in CF. From the first case report of successful pregnancy in CF in the 1960s until now, there has been a steady increase in the number of women with CF worldwide having children (Edenborough 2002). In the USA, there are now over 100 births per year for women with CF (Lyon and Bilton 2002).

There are also now reports of successful pregnancies following lung transplantation (Edenborough 2002).

There has been much concern about the potential for pregnancy to negatively affect women's health with numerous case series describing poor health outcomes following pregnancy (Cohen, di Sant'Agnese and Friedlander 1980). More recent studies suggest that with good medical care, the respiratory risks of pregnancy are minimal in women with mild, stable respiratory disease (Edenborough 2002). For those with more severe disease, pregnancy can lead to deterioration in health. Useful outcome indicators for both the mother and baby are pre-pregnancy lung function and body weight. The best outcomes are for women whose pre-pregnancy percentage predicted forced expiratory volume in one second (FEV1%) is greater than 60 per cent and pregnancy is generally not recommended for those with a pre-pregnant FEV1% of less than 50 per cent (Edenborough, Mackenzie and Stableforth 2000; Gilljam *et al.* 2000). There is, however, also a subgroup of women who experience rapid deterioration in respiratory function in pregnancy and it is difficult to know how to predict this group.

Pregnancy is best if it is planned. Edenborough (2002) recommends access to pre-conceptual genetic counselling and high-risk obstetric care, coordinated by a specialist CF service. There is little evidence of teratogenicity from maternal medications, although this always needs to be considered. Obstetric complications appear no more common than in healthy women, apart from an increased risk of pre-term delivery. This is especially related to pre-pregnancy lung function, although low body weight, the presence of CF-related diabetes mellitus, liver disease or other complications are other risk factors. Reassuringly, despite the higher proportion of pre-term deliveries there is little evidence to suggest an increase in perinatal mortality (Edenborough 2002).

Who says what, when and to whom?

The above discussion has focused on aspects of fertility and reproductive health, although as briefly discussed in the introduction, a wide range of sexual health issues are relevant to adolescents with CF. Given the risks of pregnancy, it is especially of concern that sexually active young women with CF are less likely to use contraception than otherwise healthy young women, and have erroneous beliefs about infertility and pregnancy risk (Sawyer, Phelan and Bowes 1995). It is equally of concern that approximately one in three young men with CF report confusing not needing to use contraception with not needing to protect themselves from sexually transmitted infections (Sawyer *et al.* 1998, 2005), making statements like:

> I don't need to use condoms because I don't have to worry about contraceptives.

These examples highlight the importance of ensuring that young people as well as parents have an appropriate level of knowledge and skills to protect themselves from unnecessary sexual health risks. As approximately two-thirds of adolescents and young adults want more information about sexual and reproductive health (Nixon *et al.* 2003; Sawyer *et al.* 2005), it looks like this information is not being provided. This raises the need to consider *why* these issues appear difficult to discuss, *when* these issues should be discussed and *by whom*.

In contrast to acquired medical conditions where an 'event' such as the diagnosis of cancer or the commencement of chemotherapy may act as a catalyst for a discussion of reproductive complications such as infertility, CF is a congenital condition that is generally diagnosed in infancy. In contrast to infertility as a complication of chemotherapy where actions can sometimes be taken to improve later reproductive health (e.g. egg or sperm retrieval), this is not the case in CF. Thus, while it is expected that brief discussion of likely male infertility will take place at the time of diagnosis (Sawyer and Glazner 2004), the priority of most ongoing clinic discussions with parents of children with CF is on more immediate or day-to-day CF-focused management issues.

Mothers of girls with CF report that they would like to discuss a range of sexual and reproductive health topics with their daughters' CF doctor before their daughters reach puberty (Nixon *et al.* 2003). However, this occurs uncommonly in practice (Nixon *et al.* 2003) and mothers still overwhelmingly call for more CF-specific sexual and reproductive health information to be provided. It is likely that parents of boys would be similarly interested in discussing these issues with their sons' CF doctor. However, the perspective of parents of boys with CF (both mothers and fathers) has been infrequently studied (Madge and Carr 1999; Sawyer *et al.* 1998). As with other aspects of health service delivery care, the paternal voice has been mostly absent, a research gap that deserves to be filled. For example, it is not known whether in relationship to sexual and reproductive health, fathers may wish to play a larger role in these discussions with their sons or daughters than they might in other aspects of CF care.

When should health professionals commence discussions with young people themselves? Both young men and women report wanting to discuss the sexual and reproductive health complications of CF from early adolescence. In practice, however, discussions with health professionals commonly occur later. For example, young men generally find out about male infertility two years later than they would like to (the mean age reported to first hear about male infertility was 16 years, in contrast to 14 years being the age that men thought most appropriate to first hear) (Sawyer *et al.* 1998, 2005).

Both parents and health professionals appear concerned about the effect of hearing about infertility at an early age. It is reassuring that there is no evidence that being informed about male fertility problems in CF as a young adolescent has a negative impact. Indeed, men who were first told at the age of 20 or above had a more negative reaction than men who first heard about infertility at a younger age (Sawyer *et al.* 2005). However, in younger boys, attention should be paid to language. For example, 20 per cent of adolescents reported confusing the meaning of infertility with impotence (Sawyer *et al.* 1998). For example, one teenager said:

> My mother told me I couldn't have kids but I wasn't sure what she meant, whether it was having kids or having sex.

The question of who is responsible for providing timely information and support about sexual and reproductive health in young people with CF and their families is evolving. Internationally, most speciality CF care is provided by multi-disciplinary teams, which commonly consist of physicians, nurses, physiotherapists, respiratory technicians, dieticians and social workers. In some centres, the same multi-disciplinary team cares for people from infancy through adulthood. In others, care is provided in paediatric speciality services until late adolescence or early adulthood when young people are transferred to adult speciality services. The model of care has implications for considering who is responsible for the provision of sexual and reproductive health care as well as the timing. Young people identify the specialist CF health care team as an important source of information about sexual and reproductive health (Fair *et al.* 2000; Sawyer *et al.* 1998, 2005). However, as with all elements of CF care, it is important to communicate within that team about which team members are discussing sexual and reproductive health care issues with young people and parents, to ensure these issues are being addressed.

An important prerequisite to developmentally appropriate discussions of sexual and reproductive health is health professional training. Most disciplines embodied within CF teams receive little training about the specific sexual and reproductive health aspects of CF including communication skills. Not surprisingly, CF physicians describe a number of barriers in discussing these issues with young people including insufficient training, embarrassment and difficulty finding the 'right' time for these discussions (Sawyer, Tully and Colin 2001). Other barriers are the belief that it is the parents' responsibility and that health professionals are too busy with 'medical care' to discuss reproduction (Hull and Kass 2000). While many doctors are comfortable responding to patients' questions about sexual and reproductive health, it is important that specialist CF teams proactively initiate these discussions, as while young people want to know more, young men in particular report embarrassment when having to initiate discussions themselves (Fair *et al.* 2000; Hull and Kass 2000; Nixon *et al.* 2003).

The development of clinical guidelines would assist CF teams to better address aspects of sexual and reproductive health in young people with CF. For young men, initial discussions should include discussion of pubertal development and the basics of male fertility, highlighting the distinction between infertility and impotence and the importance of preventing sexually transmitted infections. Discussions with older adolescents should include the offer of semen analysis and provide more information on assisted reproductive options – discussions that need to be repeated with young adults. For young women with CF, initial discussions about sexual and reproductive health should include pubertal development, urinary incontinence and recurrent vaginal yeast infections, normal fertility and the need to prevent unplanned pregnancy and sexually transmitted infections. Over time, pregnancy risks need to be reviewed, reinforcing the importance of pregnancy planning.

Written information is viewed by young people as a useful source of information (Fair *et al.* 2000; Sawyer *et al.* 2005) and the development of patient-oriented resources is to be encouraged. An example of a sexual and reproductive health resource that has been specially developed for young people with CF can be viewed electronically at http://www.rch.org.au/emplibrary/cah/What_they_dont_tell_you.pdf.

Genetic and ethical considerations

Both genetic and ethical issues need to be considered when discussing these issues with young people with CF and their families. They need to be kept in mind with adolescents as much as adults, as the expectations and attitudes that are formed about future relationships and parenting roles can be as much refined through the lens of what is said or left unsaid in health consultations, as they are more dominantly formed by family and culture.

All children of people affected by CF will at least be CF carriers, but the risk of having a child with CF depends on the carrier status of the non-CF partner. If the non-CF partner is tested and known not to be a carrier, the risk of CF in any children is very low (but not zero, due to the possibility of there being a CF mutation that is undetected on screening). In the uncommon situation where the non-CF partner is found to be a carrier, there is a 50 per cent chance that each pregnancy will be homozygous[4] for CF. In this situation, antenatal diagnosis using chorionic villus sampling can identify whether a fetus is or is not homozygous for CF, with the option of terminating an affected fetus. More recently, the use of pre-implantation genetic diagnosis with selective implantation of an unaffected fetus has also become available in some places. Other options for reproduction are the use of donor sperm or oocytes. Assisted reproductive technologies are widely available but expensive, and carry with them complex emotional and psycho-social issues. Providers of these technologies have generally taken the position that reproductive decisions are personal, with it being unethical to prohibit the use of reproductive services on social grounds (Tonelli 1997).

Not all people with CF would consider the possibility of having a child with CF unacceptable, an issue that obviously needs to be dealt with sensitively. To assume that parents would choose to terminate an affected fetus could be interpreted as devaluing the life of the person with CF being counselled (Tonelli 1997). A French study reported that of 64 children born to women with CF, four had inherited CF. In two of these four, the parents had chosen not to have antenatal testing undertaken (Gillet et al. 2002). However, the use of genetic technologies varies widely between different populations. For example, in the situation where couples have a child with CF and have a subsequent pregnancy, 66 per cent of Australian women used prenatal diagnosis and chose to terminate 10 of the 12 affected pregnancies (Dudding et al. 2000). Thirty-four per cent of French couples opted for prenatal diagnosis, terminating 100 per cent of affected pregnancies (Scotet et al. 2000). In contrast, 21 per cent of American couples used prenatal

diagnosis, of which 100 per cent were carried to term, including three pregnancies (one-third of cases) where CF was diagnosed (Mischler *et al.* 1998).

A central aspect of reproductive counselling in people with CF is the
consideration of the reduced life expectancy of the parent with CF and the
resultant emotional, financial and psychological effects (Tonelli 1997). The
prognosis of the affected parent needs to be discussed objectively with both
partners to ensure that both are fully informed. In many countries, the age
that women are having their first child is now older than in previous generations. This has significant implications for young women with CF whose
lung function generally worsens with age.

Summary

Young people with CF face the same array of sexual and reproductive health
issues as otherwise healthy young people, but face additional sexual and
reproductive health issues that are specific to CF. The focus here has been on
fertility and the management of reproduction, but could equally have
focused on other sexual and reproductive health complications of CF, such
as vaginal yeast infections and urinary incontinence.

While there have been significant advances in our knowledge and management of various sexual and reproductive health complications in young
people with CF, there is still much scope for improvement in health care services to ensure that young people and their families are sensitively informed
about these issues in a developmentally appropriate and timely manner. Too
often, the discomfort and embarrassment that is felt by health professionals
when discussing sexual and reproductive health topics result in the relative
invisibility of these issues within CF consultations. Embarrassment is likely
to be compounded by health professionals downplaying the importance of
topics not associated with active disease as is reported to occur when health
professional training and expertise is focused on disease control with less
emphasis on emotional, socio-cultural and developmental aspects of illness
(Sharp, Struss and Lorch 1992). Both these elements risk the future sexual
health and well-being of young people with CF.

Young people with CF and their parents want to know how sexual and
reproductive health is affected by CF and they wish to hear this in a timely
manner. Ensuring that health professionals are fully informed about these
issues and know how best to discuss them as a standard element of CF care
is a priority, as these issues are too important to ignore.

Notes

1 Not sex-linked.
2 Chronic, abnormal dilation of the bronchi, causing a persistent productive cough and recurring infections.
3 Structure within the scrotum that stores, matures and transports sperm.
4 Having identical alleles (one member of pair) for a single trait.

12.

Dispelling the Taboo
of Intersex Conditions
We're Only Human Like You!

Melissa Cull

Introduction

Congenital Adrenal Hyperplasia (CAH) (also referred to as Adrenogenital Syndrome [AGS]) is one of a number of so-called intersex conditions in which the individual can show anatomical characteristics of both sexes. This chapter draws on available research, illustrated by personal and support group experiences, to consider the issues arising from moving through adolescence to adulthood while living with conditions that have the potential to be shrouded in secrecy and stigma. Many of the experiences contained here are equally applicable to those living with other intersex and associated conditions such as Androgen Insensitivity Syndrome (AIS),[1] Swyer's Syndrome,[2] true hermaphroditism (see below), Mayer-Rokitansky-Kuster-Hauser Syndrome (MRKH),[3] and vaginal hypoplasia,[4] though CAH is one of the only intersex conditions that is life-threatening.

CAH is a rare (1:10,000) life-threatening autosomal recessive genetic condition (see Chapter 4). It affects the adrenal glands' production of cortisol and salt-retaining hormones and can result in a life-threatening adrenal crisis. The block in the production of cortisol and the enzyme 21 Hydroxylase or 11 Beta, and the resulting excess production of androgens (sex hormones), often causes virilization of females or, in a very rare number of cases such as with StAR CAH, feminization of males. At birth, the female's external genitals can appear to be male, for example showing cliteromegaly (enlarged clitoris), fused labia and a mis-positioned vaginal opening often fused with the urethra (pseudohermaphroditism). The fused labia and enlarged clitoris can resemble a small scrotum and penis or, more ambiguously, appear neither male nor female. CAH is therefore a pheno-typical intersex condition in that the external genitalia appear to be male yet internal reproductive organs are functionally female and chromosomes XX or vice versa for males with, for example, StAR CAH. True herma-phroditism is where both ovarian and testicular cells are present. Intersex conditions have been reported to affect 2 per cent of the world's population or 1 in 50 families (Diamond 2000).

There are several different types of CAH, ranging from salt-wasting, non-salt-wasting and simple virilizing types (which require steroid replace-ment), to milder late onset non-virilizing CAH (which sometimes does not). Cortisol and salt-retaining hormones must be replaced with lifelong steroid treatment; such treatment only being possible since the mid-1950s and only achieving better standards of success more recently. CAH is more difficult to detect in males as there are often no visible outward effects. Failure to thrive can be one of the indicators and, in the past, boys tended to die in early infancy. However, males typically have milder symptoms, mainly height and weight related as a result of steroid treatment.

For later onset CAH, both females and males can enter precocious puberty from two to four years of age (see Chapter 4). This can be controlled medically but may result in short stature. However, affected children are often much taller and more physically developed than their peers in the early stages and this can lead to teasing and bullying. Some adult males in particular have identified this in support groups as a source of great distress.

Having ambiguous genitalia can be traumatic to the growing child and adolescent. Some males report above-average penis size and an increase in libido as a result of excess testosterone. Although this is experienced posi-tively by some, others report negative impact through greater mood swings and aggression. Most females require surgery at some stage to unfuse the labia, separate the vagina from the urethra and reposition the opening (vaginoplasty). The most highly controversial type of surgery is clitoral reduction or clitoral recession or clitorectomy (clitoral amputation – sup-posedly now only rarely performed in the UK but still practised widely in some countries). Clitoral surgery (clitoroplasty) can lead to sexual dysfunc-tion, loss of sensate function and inability to achieve orgasm (Crouch et al. 2004; Minto et al. 2003). Clitororectomy is basically the same surgical procedure as female genital mutilation (FGM) practised by some religions and cultures. Although it has been illegal to perform FGM in the UK since 1985, no such laws protect the intersexed female.

'Normalizing surgery', as it is known, is almost entirely carried out in early infancy (before the age of two) despite the fact that a vagina is not required until menstruation starts at puberty. Medically speaking, vagino-plasty may be required earlier than puberty if urinary stones form and cause infection, though this is rare (Balen *et al.* 2004). It appears that parents and doctors, perhaps influenced by societal pressures, find it difficult to accept genital ambiguity. Concerns about parents' ability to bond with their child and the child's psycho-sexual development are also cited as reasons for early surgery (Berenbaum and Bailey 2003; Warne *et al.* 2005). However, surgery is permanent and potentially damaging (Minto, Creighton and Woodhouse 2001). And with increasing awareness of the range of difference in the appearance of genitalia among women who do not have intersex conditions (Blank 1993) the desire to achieve a so-called normal appearance appears even more outdated.

As girls mature, surgery is often required to facilitate menstruation, tampon use and sexual intercourse (BAPS 2001; Creighton 2001; Creighton and Minto 2001; Creighton, Minto and Steele 2001; Creighton *et al.* 2002; Crouch *et al.* 2004). It is therefore crucial that they are kept informed in an age-appropriate way of their condition and its treatment (including surgical interventions) and involved in decision-making (Carmichael and Alderson 2004; MacDougall 2004) (for a fuller discussion see Chapter 7).

Sexual function is reported to be impaired in over 85 per cent of women with CAH who have had surgery regardless of whether this has been carried out in infancy or later, though the research on the latter is limited (Creighton *et al.* 2001, 2002; Crouch *et al.* 2004). Sexual function is also impaired to a lesser extent in those that have not had surgery. The degree to which surgery proves psychologically damaging is not well researched but support groups hear from professionals as well as affected individuals about how devastated teenagers and young adults are when they find out this has happened to them as young children without their consent (Creighton and Minto 2001).

For males, providing they take their medications correctly throughout life and check regularly for testicular adrenal rests (adrenal tissue that comes to rest in other areas of the body such as the testicles and may lead to their calcification or, in rare instances, testicular cancer), fertility is usually not impaired. If adrenal rests *are* found and appropriate medication prescribed, male CAH infertility is often reversible. Fertility is reduced by 80–90 per cent for women with salt-wasting CAH and by 20–40 per cent for those with the non-salt-wasting/simple virilizing/late onset types. Females often have fertility problems even with the milder forms of CAH that do not virilize. Indeed, investigation for fertility difficulties and also hirsutism (excess hairiness) is a common route through which late or adult onset CAH is diagnosed. It is very common for all women with CAH, especially those with the salt-wasting forms, to have polycystic ovary syndrome (PCOS) due to excess exposure to pre-natal (in the womb) androgens (see Chapter 4). However, given that pregnancy is not without health risks, it is important that good contraceptive advice from a gynaecologist and endocrinologist is available to avoid unplanned pregnancies in those women who are fertile.

As a last resort, radical bilateral adrenalectomy (removal of both adrenal glands) can be performed, though this is not without controversy. For some women and also men with medically uncontrolled CAH or excessive obesity resulting from CAH treatment, this 'cures' the CAH by stopping the production of excess androgens. However, the down side is that it is not without risk and fatalities or complications have resulted in some cases. It can also increase longer-term mortality risks as the resulting steroid replacement treatment is for life and dosages must be increased during any illness. Any cessation of treatment, even if brief, can result in death within 24 hours so it is not a suitable option for anyone who is, or at risk of being, non-compliant with treatment. On the positive side, female fertility and weight in both sexes have been reported to improve following bilateral adrenalectomy. Recently, one woman with salt-wasting CAH known to the AHN (Adrenal Hyperplasia Network) support group, who had tried for a number of years to conceive without success despite many different infertility interventions, was successful in having a live birth only after a radical bilateral adrenalectomy.

Coping with treatment and its long-term effects is an important aspect of living with CAH. At whatever stage it is diagnosed, it is important to remember that conditions that can have associated sexual differentiation and developmental problems are shrouded in shame and secrecy. Nondisclosure is high and those affected can experience lack of self-esteem, poor body image and social isolation.

My experience of living and coping with CAH

As a female with salt-wasting CAH, growing up was quite traumatic. My parents knew very little, as doctors had simply told them I would need steroid replacement for life in order to stay alive and that they could 'fix me surgically' for the genital ambiguity. While doctors were allowed to examine, poke and prod intimate parts of my body, no explanation was given to me other than 'Take the tablets, have the surgery, don't ask questions, don't tell anyone anything and don't touch, everything will be OK.' In reality it has been far from OK. I became very shy and withdrawn. While my peers always seemed to have lots of friends, went out and so on, I stayed in, had few friends and felt unable to talk to them. I was forever in and out of hospital and had endless hospital visits for check-ups. The surgery was very traumatic.

Age 4

Total clitorectomy. My enlarged clitoris of two to three cm did not bother me or cause pain. Following surgery, I had lots of pain and heavy scarring and was always told not to look at or touch my body. I was extremely frightened as I was well when I went into hospital and came out feeling ill with a huge sense of loss, even though at the time I did not know what had been done to me, or what the significance was going to be later in life. I just knew that something was missing. I went from being a happy child, although quite sickly, to being withdrawn.

Age 11

First vaginoplasty. Again no explanation other than 'Something's not quite right and the doctor will fix it. Don't ask questions.' As I was just into puberty, this was traumatic with a gynaecologist poking and prodding intimate parts of me followed by surgery.

Age 12

Told at check-up that I would never be able to have children. I was totally devastated and became more withdrawn. I was also told that if I wanted to marry I would need to see a gynaecologist before doing so and not to ever let anyone, especially men, see my body except for doctors. The surgery is supposed to make a female with CAH more 'visually' and physically acceptable sexually to men and to enable 'married life', which I later realized was a euphemism for sexual intercourse.

Age 13

More surgery as the first vaginoplasty had scarred and developed stenosis (scarring that causes surrounding tissue to shrink) and had adhesions (small pieces of tissue that had stuck to the sides of the repaired vagina). No one had explained to me at the time why surgical packing had been placed inside me or why there was lots of blood so I had pulled the packing out as it was agonisingly painful. This had resulted in a sharp telling off by the doctor, nurses and parents at the time and the warning that I would require more surgery as a result. The final surgery was to remove the adhesions and widen the vaginal opening.

Age 14

Dilatation treatment. Six weeks after the final surgery, I was introduced to dilatation. Dilators at this time were glass, similar to test tubes but stronger. They were coned, phallic-shaped instruments graduating from quite small to 'average male' size. The experience was very traumatic and not how dilatation should be done. The doctor roughly inserted the dilator into the barely healed vaginal opening then removed it and repeated the process a number of times. I was told to go away and do this three times daily for ten minutes a time 'for the rest of your life or until you get married'. No explanation was offered as to why or what for. It felt more like abuse than medical treatment. My parents were horrified and thought it was a form of masturbation rather than a medical treatment to prevent the surgically repaired vaginal opening from collapsing and shrinking back to pre-surgery state. So they did not encourage me to do the dilatation exercises. There was no privacy and anyway I was worried the dilators would break. I'd always been told never to touch my body so having to touch and insert dilators into the very parts of my body that had always been a total taboo proved difficult. I was also worried I would need more horrific surgery. I rarely did the treatment as I felt disgusted and frightened. I felt a total lack of body ownership. When I returned for check-ups I would be told off for not doing them and no counselling or support was ever provided.

Age 18

I found a support group that covered many metabolic conditions including CAH. On reading the information sent, I felt such relief to not be alone, to learn what CAH was, the meaning of intersex and the basics of what the surgery was. I felt a great stone had lifted. Prior to then, I had thought I must have cancer. Being told I could die if I was ill and/or did not take the medication and always being in and out of hospital without explanations, I thought the worst: that it was something so bad that the doctors could never tell me. I felt a mixture of anger and sadness as well as great relief, now knowing I could live as long as anyone else providing I sought prompt medical treatment when ill to avoid life-threatening adrenal crisis. Anger that nobody had explained CAH and the intersex aspects and sadness that I had missed out on my childhood. From that point onwards, I came to understand more clearly than before that many of the difficulties that I had experienced were to do with the way that my condition had been reacted to rather than to do with me.

Managing adult sexual relationships

Growing up, I had few friends and little social interaction. CAH can affect your social life both through its impact on self-esteem, body image and confidence but also through the necessity, for some, for frequent hospital visits and in-patient stays simply to stay well and alive. Like any teenager, I had begun to have sexual feelings but was too scared and frightened to explore them. So, while my friends and peers seemed to be getting on with their lives and having boyfriends, I avoided the issue, shut off and suppressed feelings, got on with my schooling and then work. I felt isolated and lonely and lacked confidence around people – a very common experience for those with CAH (May, Boyle and Grant 1996). I wondered how anyone could love or want me, thought that I could not reciprocate and felt a failure – though more failed by society and doctors as surgery made me look worse than 'nature's mistakes'.

Libido is another unknown. For many women it can range from 'low' to 'high'. With CAH this is also true but excess testosterone and androgens can, for some, cause libido to be very high. CAH can thus be a 'treble-edged sword': it can be life-threatening, result in surgical damage to genitalia (particularly the clitoris) and cause high libido. Anorgasmia (inability to reach orgasm), dyspareunia (pain on sexual intercourse) and sexual frustration are often reported.

With the body's 'hormonal soup' being disturbed by CAH, stress is also common, as is depression in both females and males. Socialization and the ability to emotionally bond may also be impeded, as recent research has suggested that the brain's amygdala may be affected through pre-natal hormones (Merke *et al.* 2003).

As I got older and my friends gradually paired off, settled down, married and started to have children, my 'body clock' started ticking and I wondered if I would ever meet anyone who would accept me. I did meet someone in my twenties and we had a relationship but he found it difficult to accept what CAH was and the damage the surgery had caused so, after a few years, we split up. Instead of bringing us closer together, sex drove us further apart. While most people experience pleasure, I was just experiencing pain, both physical and emotional. Painkillers were no use as then I was completely numb and felt nothing at all. If I did not take them, despite my partner being very gentle whenever we had sexual intercourse, I would feel nothing but intense physical pain and would sit with tears streaming down my face, which did neither of us any good. I felt emotional pain too: I had been brought up to believe that only doctors could ever touch me, so when I fell in love I felt it was wrong for my boyfriend to touch me and would get vivid flashbacks to gynaecological examinations.

I consulted my GP but his only advice was 'use it or lose it' (meaning that the surgically repaired vagina was shrinking) so I asked for a referral to a gynaecologist. By the time I got a referral it was too late, the relationship was failing and the female gynaecologist I saw, although nice, had no experience of CAH. I was told to persevere and to take painkillers.

I still had little explanation as to what exactly had been done to me or why. I felt a failure as a woman, but also felt 'at least it is better to have loved and lost than never to have loved at all'. I just threw myself back into work and studies to forget.

My experience of gynaecologists and surgical outcomes is not uncommon, including among younger women of today, and many relate similar experiences to the AHN support group. Others are too frightened to enter into relationships for fear of rejection or the need for further surgery. However, some do find caring, understanding partners and go on to gain some pleasure from sexual activities despite pain, emotional upset and compromised ability to achieve orgasm.

Coming together – the value of support groups

Meeting other people with CAH and other intersex conditions was a great help. Realizing that the majority of people with intersex conditions had similar experiences to me, with the same lack of information, inspired me to do support work. Knowledge is the key to understanding and coping. I worked voluntarily for many years with CLIMB (Children Living with Inherited MetaBolic Diseases) and CAHG (CAH Support Group of CLIMB) before founding AHN (Adrenal Hyperplasia Network – www.ahn.org.uk) in 1999. AHN works with professionals and researchers, as well as other support groups such as Androgen Insensitivity Syndrome Support Group (AISSG), Rokitansky Support and Advice (ROSA) and Genetic Interest Group (GIG), to improve treatment and provide support to people of all ages, although we focus on teenagers and adults. Doing this also inspired me to change career from being a quality engineer to researcher. I turned the negatives on their head so they became positives.

Growing up can be difficult enough for teenagers. With intersex conditions, it can be made even more difficult when there are few, if any, information or emotional support services available and limited empathy in professional encounters. Support groups can be a great help to parents, children, teenagers and adults in providing much needed information about the condition itself and its treatment, meeting with others and sharing experiences in a safe environment. Knowing you are not alone can make an enormous difference. Professionals too can learn a great deal from support groups.

Increasingly, professionals are realizing the importance of careful preparation, counselling and support to those affected and their parents and family members at all life stages – yet more needs to be done and to be available more consistently. The AHN support group provides consultation and advice to professionals and works with them to produce patient-friendly information sheets. Members provide input to professional training, including through contributing to medical training films and speaking at conferences as well as providing a direct service to those affected and their families through website, telephone, email and written support as well as individual and face-to-face meetings.

However, there is also a need for challenges to be made to the way that intersex conditions are perceived at a societal level – changing attitudes from childhood onwards, including, for example, through sex education, by promoting awareness and dispelling myths. AHN is thus involved in the

Expert Patients initiative (available at www.doh.gov.uk) as well as media work (Melton 2001).

Living in Western society where sex, sexuality and perfection command high media attention, having a stigmatized condition like CAH is not easy. Intersexism is rife in almost all cultures and this makes it particularly difficult for people to speak publicly about their experiences and be assured of an understanding reception. At a personal level, this means that telling a partner about the outcome of surgery that was done as a child – especially when the main intention of this was to make you more socially acceptable – is difficult and distressing. Sexual disability remains a taboo subject, rarely discussed and highly stigmatized. Discussion of the human rights aspects remains at a preliminary level and 'champions' are thin on the ground – yet people living with intersex have feelings, wants and needs like anyone else (Cull 2002).

Despite the majority view of sex/sexuality being bipolar – male or female – the reality is that it is more of a continuum as we are increasingly coming to realize (Blackless *et al.* 2000). Genital ambiguity is therefore simply one end of the continuum. Consider the difference to society if the continuum was acknowledged, where children would be spared the stigma that is currently attached to intersex conditions and where any health and psycho-social interventions were truly person-centred.

However, there is another risk to living with intersex conditions. Being 'different' can invite unwanted attention from caregivers, relatives, health professionals and religious groups. Support groups and professionals hear an increasing number of complaints from their members about sexual, mental and physical abuse. Sexual abuse can range from curiosity to full-blown sexual assaults. Mental and physical abuse can occur at the hands of those few caregivers who cannot cope, accept or understand, so see their child as a 'freak' and treat them as such. Knowing how, when and who to trust can be very difficult for us.

The way ahead

I felt totally 'medicalized', with a total lack of body ownership, until I got a third opinion on surgery at 31 years of age. Only then, with counselling and support, did I learn to be able to cope better. The original male gynaecologist had been abrupt, 'old school' and intimidating. The second opinion gynaecologist was female and more caring but did not understand CAH and was of little help. The third opinion gynaecologist and her specialist registrar, both female, were extremely caring, empathic and understanding of CAH. On examining me, these two doctors were themselves almost brought to tears even though they were specialists in the field. For me, to experience the doctors expressing some visible emotions was such a relief.

Being told that there was nothing more surgically that could be done to reduce the scarring or to tidy up the external mess (no viable tissue was left) unless and until there were medical advances with stem cell research was extremely upsetting. However, to be told that the internal surgery was OK and 'functional' was a relief, even though the knowledge that sensate function was severely damaged or impaired and that pain on sexual intercourse was something I would have to live with was devastating. As scar tissue will always shrink and reconstructed vaginas are not as stretchy or flexible as natural ones, renewed dilatation treatment was recommended. This time, treatment was with unbreakable plastic dilators and caringly demonstrated and it has, despite initial pain (eased by painkillers), stretched and relieved much of the stenosis. Initially for 30 minutes three times daily for three months, over time it was reduced to three times a week. Surgery is not the 'one stage fix' treatment it is often claimed to be and dilatation and/or regular sexual intercourse must become part of life (Creighton *et al.* 2001, 2002).

Support, counselling, time, privacy and motivation are essential to maintain dilatation treatment as it is a constant reminder of surgery and of being 'different'. Although some females are now offered it following surgery as teenagers, it is only offered to others when the possibility of sexual intercourse is imminent. However, many teenagers and women report that, unless they have a functional vagina, they will not even enter into a relationship. Others have commented to the AHN support group that they do not want to have to wait until they are in a relationship to start treatment and thereby risk losing their partner while it is set up. Many strongly object, not surprisingly, to a system that requires them to 'seek permission' to establish sexual relationships. For those with CAH who want to live a 'normal life' but who have a gynaecologist who will not routinely provide access to dilatation treatment, this can be a very vicious circle.

It is very common for members of the support group to report that a frequent comment by psychologists and doctors is that 'Sexual intercourse isn't essential to a relationship, there are other forms of sexual intimacy.' While it is true that there are indeed other forms of sexual intimacy, to have the choice taken away or severely impaired is not helpful. Women may wish to be able to give as well as receive intimacy and pleasure if they are to feel sexually whole (Liao and Boyle in press).

Regaining ownership of one's body is a very important component of ensuring that self-esteem and improved body image are restored as well as a means of avoiding the 'medicalization' of sexual function. Parents, carers and professionals need to remember that the growing child and teenager is a sexual being and will want to have similar experiences to their peers. To be told that an 'oversized clitoris is unimportant and has been removed/ reduced' despite the fact that it is the most innervated part of the woman's body (Baskin *et al.* 1999; Crouch *et al.* 2004; O'Connell *et al.* 1998) and essential for sexual pleasure is at least insensitive and at worst highly damaging. If the same was said about a man's penis there would be total outrage!

Females with CAH, as other females, express their sexual orientation as heterosexual, lesbian or bi-sexual while others report feeling that they 'don't fit' and remain asexual. Research from the USA (Meyer-Bahlburg 2001; Money, Schwartz and Lewis 1984) has suggested that an above-average number (37%) of females with CAH are lesbian, though the methodology has been challenged. More recent UK research puts the figure much lower at 5 per cent (Bainton *et al.* 1999) and this is supported by AHN support group experience. However, there is some evidence to suggest that women with CAH may be especially vulnerable to physical, sexual and mental abuse from men and that some at least have chosen same sex relationships and found greater understanding with those partners (Cull 2005; May *et al.* 1996; Morgan *et al.* 2005). The need for carers, parents and professionals to support them regardless of sexual orientation is clear.

Although many women with CAH remain single and have few sexual relationships, increasing numbers do have loving, caring, lifelong partners (May *et al.* 1996). Advances in endocrine control since the 1990s (though still not universally available), together with advances in modern fertility treatments, mean that even those with severe salt-wasting CAH have been successful in having children.

Women who have had genital surgery will require a caesarean to give birth and this may also be necessary for some who have not (Greenwell *et al.* 2003). All women with CAH need close monitoring during pregnancy to ensure that mother and baby are kept well. Pregnancies are rarely allowed to go to full term for the safety of both mother and baby. The mother will need extra steroid cover with IV steroids to avoid adrenal crisis whether or not a caesarean is performed.

As CAH is an autosomal recessive condition, the child will only have CAH if both parents have CAH. If one has CAH and the other is a carrier then the risk of transmission is 1 in 2 with the other being a carrier; if both parents are carriers then the risk reduces to 1 in 4. Between 1 in 50 and 1 in 80 of the population carry the faulty gene and increasing numbers of those with CAH are being recommended to have genetic screening as part of their family planning.

Living with CAH

Living with CAH typically means managing a lifelong regime of taking medication. Treatment with steroids affects the immune system, particularly for those with salt-wasting CAH. Even though the dose given is intended to replace the body's natural processes, it is not wholly possible. Illnesses, even those as common as flu and, in particular, diarrhoea and vomiting, chickenpox and broken limbs, can be life-threatening. If they prompt an adrenal crisis, hospitalization is required to restabilize and rehydrate the body as well as to treat the illness. People with CAH tend to be more ill with even minor conditions than those without the condition. Minor illnesses are treated with extra doses of steroids along with whatever medication the GP prescribes. Any form of surgery, including dental work, requires extra steroid cover. Hospital stays will therefore be longer as the CAH will need to be stabilized along with the medical treatment. CAH is a hidden disability so people may think you are well and perhaps over-reacting by going to the doctors with what may seem like minor ailments. Schools, colleges and employers need to be aware that you have to attend the doctor or hospital more frequently as well as knowing what needs to be done in an emergency.

Most people with salt-wasting CAH carry emergency steroid injections, which help them buy enough time to get to hospital and start on IV fluids in order to avoid adrenal crisis. Adrenal crisis is frightening and indescribable to those who have never experienced it. Steroid cards, CAH info cards and instructions as to what to do in an emergency should be carried. As well as illness, stress can also bring on adrenal crisis so caregivers, schools, colleges and employers need to be aware of this. Overall, however, there are few restrictions on what a person with CAH can do.

As a child with severe salt-wasting CAH, I was often ill and in and out of hospital but, thankfully, this is less frequent now I am an adult. Frequent hospital admissions are stressful for the person affected and their family especially when other family members, friends and colleagues find them difficult to understand. Situations where there is the risk of infection have to be avoided. It may not be possible to organize much in advance and plans sometimes have to be changed at short notice either because of illness or danger of exposure to infections.

'Getting a life' can be difficult but is far from impossible. It takes determination and a good support network of family, caregivers and friends together with well-informed doctors to keep you physically and emotionally well. As for me, I am now 37 years old. I hold down a very interesting career working as a research assistant to a consultant diabetologist/endocrinologist, study part-time for a psychology degree and have wide-ranging interests in my social life. I am the founder of AHN, working at promoting awareness and improving treatment. I am not ashamed to have an intersex condition; it is simply part of who I am. My experiences of living with CAH are, sadly, still being replicated today in children and young people growing up with an intersex condition and my story and those of others needs to be told so that the lessons can be learnt. My experiences have enabled me to understand other people better, especially those living with adversity. Who knows what the future will bring – perhaps marriage and children, fertility permitting – but the work to lift the taboo of intersex goes on.

Notes

1 Where a person has a functioning Y sex chromosome, but the X sex chromosome has an abnormality that causes the body to be incapable of recognizing the androgens (male hormones) produced. As a result the person has some or all of the physical characteristics of a woman, despite having the genetic makeup of a man.
2 Where a person has a normal vagina and uterus but has no ovaries or testes.
3 Characterized by an absent or incomplete vagina, an incompletely developed uterus, but normal fallopian tubes and ovaries.
4 Where at least the upper third of the vagina is missing, common in AIS.

13.

Sexuality and Growing Up HIV-Positive
Lessons from Practice

Nancy Cincotta, Jocelyn Childs and Andrew Eichenfield

Introduction

Children born HIV-positive who are ageing into adolescence and young adulthood are a unique, emerging population. The issue of their sexuality is an uncharted domain. Never before has there been a group of teenagers and young adults who acquired HIV perinatally and who have lived long enough to have reached the complicated period of normal development that includes experimentation with sexual activity and managing the choices involved in long-term relationships and childbearing. Never again will there be a population in this particular situation, born to a group of caregivers unprepared to deal with the immediate and long-term issues of the then new HIV epidemic at a time when there was less hope for the survival of an HIV-positive child.

The focus of this chapter is derived from, and illustrated by, clinical work with children and young people who were perinatally infected with HIV. Their HIV-related medical and mental health care was initiated when they were infants and toddlers. Of primary concern in the early years of the AIDS epidemic was the high mortality rate. From a medical standpoint and in the minds of caregivers, there was an expectation that children who were HIV-positive would have a short life. As the nature of the epidemic has changed, so have circumstances surrounding the medical care, the ways children learn they are infected and the responses of those around them. Disclosure of HIV status generally and disclosing to individual children who are affected has been a dominant concern for caregivers and health care providers in the past two decades (Lipson 1993; Tasker 1992; Wiener, Battles and Heilman 1998). Whom to tell, what to tell and when to tell have been well researched and are very familiar issues for those professionals who work with people with HIV (Ledlie 1999).

For this particular group of children and young people, their entire lives have been affected by the challenges of coping with HIV, a condition that has taken two decades to better understand and treat. The legacy of the AIDS epidemic is integrated into the emotional framework of those living with HIV. For the most part, children who were perinatally infected have (or indeed have not) learned about their condition in a variety of ways. Their lives carry with them the same uncertainty about the future that they have carried since birth.

Medical advances have allowed for the early recognition and treatment of HIV and for a much more positive outlook on longer-term survival. Developmental issues that impose challenges for families in which there are no underlying medical conditions impose themselves equally on the lives of HIV-positive youth. In the course of routine development, children, by the time they reach adolescence, begin to establish a perception of themselves and their future. It is common for them to see all things as being possible and within reach (Erikson 1950). Many young adults will not have experienced loss and, for those that have, it is often the loss of a grandparent.

The perceptions of the future of HIV-positive teens and young adults are challenged by what they believe their life course will be, what they know about those family members who are affected or who have died of HIV and the reality of their medical situation. In the United States, in addition to the realistic facts of their own situation (minority ethnic groups and socio-economically disadvantaged groups are affected disproportionately by HIV/AIDS), teens and young adults must live in a society that infrequently embraces those who are HIV-positive. The honesty with which a teen or young adult approaches relationships with others will be influenced by a myriad of circumstances, often based on the individual's past experiences. The experience of their own HIV status, how they perceive that their HIV-positive family members have been treated, the outcomes of each family member's illness and what their family relationships have been like will all influence their actions on facing their first and subsequent physical and emotional relationships.

The course of the lives of children who are HIV-positive

This particular group of children and young people have lived during two very different times. Initially there was a sentiment that children should not know their diagnosis. This was because society had not made peace with the idea of children diagnosed with a condition that was both potentially infectious and life-threatening. Currently there is more of a focus on informing children of their diagnosis (American Academy of Pediatrics 1999) and research suggests the benefits to the child and family of disclosing the information to others (Sherman *et al.* 2000; Wiener, Battles and Heilman 2000). Disclosure, however, remains a complicated issue as it impacts on the child's experience in school and in the community. There is still a pervasive stigma surrounding the diagnosis (Herek and Glunt 1988; Herek, Capitanio and Widamen 2003). Once children who are HIV-positive come to understand their HIV status, the issues then include how they involve others with information about their diagnosis and treatment. The decisions they make, who they make them with and the dialogues they engage in are all part of this uncharted journey in which these children, not always with the strongest of social supports and resources, are forging ahead. It is a challenge for the professionals from whom these youth receive their care to join them on their journey and to try to help them make sense of it along the way. A recent study of HIV-positive adolescents noted that the majority were sexually active and almost half of the cohort reported unprotected sex at last intercourse. Higher levels of depression were associated with unprotected sex and alcohol use (Murphy *et al.* 2001).

Not the purview of the paediatrician

Coming to recognize HIV-positive youth as sexually interested and active imposes a struggle for both health and mental health providers in paediatrics:

> A 12-year-old denied any interest in sex when talking to her doctor. The team was taken by surprise when they received a call from the school saying the 12-year-old was found having oral sex with a peer. Perhaps due to their own discomfort or disbelief that children should be sexually active, providers may overlook or deny signs that suggest children are

developing into adolescents. There develops a partnership in disbelief that protects both parties from having to talk about something uncomfortable.

When professionals are involved in providing care for young children, often from birth, they become connected to the child and the progress that they make as they grow and achieve normal developmental milestones. They have long-term relationships with these children and their families, become comfortable and, in many ways, feel a bit like 'family'. What component of professional training prepares the health and social work team for children growing up and becoming sexually active? Making the transition to seeing them in this light, especially when their engagement in sexual activity starts young, can be challenging.

Many professionals did not enter into taking care of children with HIV by plan. Older clinicians (those who studied in the 1950s, 1960s and early 1970s) trained before HIV was even a known entity or component of training in paediatric infectious diseases. Those who trained in the 1980s and early 1990s did so at a time when HIV in children was seen as a terminal illness. For this professional cohort, the relationships children would develop in later life were not the primary focus. Switching gears and growing to understand who these children are and will be as young adults represents a paradigm shift both for those focused on 'paediatric care' and those who have had decades of experience with HIV-positive children. Providers do not necessarily easily change their way of thinking about those with whom they work.

Children and young people who are HIV-positive: the journey forward

Studies show children with perinatal HIV infections who are ageing into adolescence are typically healthy and may have no outward symptoms of the disease (Thorne *et al.* 2002). The majority are on several medications (*ibid.*) and must confront the difficulties of adherence to a complex medical regimen. They tend to be a heterogeneous group in terms of drug history and sexual history; despite their health condition, they are like their HIV-negative counterparts in that they are vulnerable to risky behaviour (Frederick *et al.* 2000). The normal challenges of adolescence – sexuality, experimentation and independence – must all be addressed within the context of HIV (Ledlie 2001).

Whereas there is much literature on disclosure of HIV status to children and adolescents (Ledlie 1999; Sherman *et al.* 2000; Wiener *et al.* 2000), little has been written about the emerging sexuality of the HIV-positive child. What young people who are HIV-positive feel and experience as they approach stages in life in which they must make decisions about themselves that have an impact on others has had limited exploration. It is not well documented that many clinicians are in discussion with HIV-positive children about their relationships and their choices:

> How should teenagers express to another teen that they are HIV-positive? Should they always disclose? When should they disclose? At the beginning of a friendship? After trust has developed? If this is someone with whom the adolescent thinks they will have a more physical relationship, should they tell the other person they are HIV-positive before they progress to a closer relationship? Should this be discussed before any physical contact? Before sexual contact? What are the implications for the youth who is HIV-positive and what are the implications for the potential partner? What happens when the teen invariably 'breaks up' with the person to whom they have disclosed? Are the rules different for adults or for teens? What information sharing is in the best interest of whom?

Mental health professionals at the forefront of medical care are in a position to assess and address these questions as part of the routine care of children and young people who are HIV-positive. Studies suggest that teens do not plan to become sexually active, it just 'happens' (Brooks-Gunn and Furstenberg 1989). This indicates a need for providers to pre-emptively initiate a dialogue about sex.

At an age when youth often find themselves in a series of relationships there are complicated issues that emerge. Once an individual discloses their HIV status to a peer, they cannot go back and 'undisclose' the information. The choice to disclose in a relationship that may be temporary is emotionally laden. The *first* disclosure to a friend, peer, boyfriend or girlfriend could be the *last* disclosure. Young teenagers may not always be mature in their ability to discern the strengths, weaknesses and trustworthiness of their peers. As a result, such decisions are complex and cumbersome:

> In one situation, a father decided it was time to tell his 14-year-old daughter that she was HIV-positive. She had been having sex with a

14-year-old friend at school (unbeknownst to her father). In response to the information that she was HIV-positive, and in an attempt to be responsible, she told her boyfriend that she had just learned she was HIV-positive. He panicked and told the principal, who panicked and called the police. Both children were suspended from school and suddenly everyone in the school knew that this child was HIV-positive.

Differentiating issues for behaviourally affected teens

Although not the focus of this chapter, it is unclear whether there has ever been a study comparing *behaviourally* infected children and *perinatally* infected children with regard to issues around self-esteem, disclosure, sexual relationships or childbearing. Youth who are behaviourally infected have known life before being HIV-positive. Some of their views and actions may be strongly influenced by their experience of growing up HIV-negative. There may be differences in the perceptions of those who are perinatally infected versus those who are behaviourally infected. For instance, in order to have been behaviourally infected in the first world, the individual concerned had to be (knowingly or unknowingly) exposed to drug use or a sexual relationship or abuse.

While many life stressors may be the same for the two populations (including those arising from both groups containing disproportionately high numbers from minority ethnic and socio-economically disadvantaged backgrounds), there is inherently a difference resulting from a lifetime of feeling burdened by taking medications and coping with an incurable health condition. For those perinatally infected, the experience is similar to growing up with a genetic or chronic illness that you have had your entire life. You are connected to an 'illness' community and you share some component of the 'illness' with others of the family into which you were born.

Developmental issues

Finding one's place in society and the exploration of one's sexuality is a natural component of adolescent development, yet it is a period that can be complicated emotionally. The process is further exacerbated when an adolescent or young adult is HIV-positive. Teenagers, consistent with their development, will be impulsive and caught up with their own confusing emotions. Even the demands that one carries because of an HIV diagnosis may not mitigate against a teen's natural inclinations. One study showed that a history of a past STD diagnosis was associated with increased prevention knowledge but not with motivation to use protection (DiClemente *et al.* 2002). In fact, adolescents with a history of a diagnosed infection were more likely to report *not* using a condom at most recent intercourse, suggesting that teens are not applying learned knowledge to their current sexual behaviour. All the discussion, planning and processing of how a youth who is HIV-positive might approach a relationship or a sexual encounter may be set aside when peer pressure and their own need to 'belong' enter the formula.

As children age into adolescence and young adulthood, they begin to identify themselves in ways in which they are similar to, and different from, their parents. For a child who is HIV-positive and whose parent is, or was, HIV-positive, these issues carry another layer of ambiguity. If you are HIV-positive through perinatal transmission, then at least one, and often both, of your parents are, or were, HIV-positive. You may feel more connected to that parent and feel that you share the burden but also the commonality of HIV/AIDS. Alternatively, you may feel anger and resentment that HIV was transmitted to you. Some families may adapt, united by their family battle against HIV/AIDS. Others may disintegrate, unable to respond to the overwhelming challenges.

The reality of the involvement of many family members differentiates HIV from other conditions. Parents, who are often pivotal in the development of identity for evolving youth, may be less available because of the severity of their own illness. When a parent dies of AIDS and their child is in the custody of another caregiver, the child may be subjected to a preconceived notion about their sexuality, tainted by the awareness that their parent died of HIV. This knowledge, consciously or unconsciously, may influence the caregiver's perceptions of how children, teens and young adults who are HIV-positive should act. The family issues surrounding grief and bereavement also play a role in how children and young people who are HIV-positive see themselves in relationship to their parents, their health status and the world.

Secrets

Growing up HIV-positive may bring its own culture. In many families, there has been a history of less than open communication about HIV. These secrets became part of their culture early on as parents were dying of AIDS and their children were placed in the custody of others. Particularly in the case of younger HIV-positive children, there was a sense that, as they were not going to live and would not understand, they did not need to be burdened by the painful details of their parent's illness. In other words, these secrets were not initiated by the children. Yet, when children grow up in such an environment, keeping secrets becomes a skill and a way of being that is learned. Under normal circumstances, children will often hide things from their parents. In this case, information was hidden from the child and so a pattern was already begun, placing this population at unusual and unfortunate risk. Now we are expecting teens who may want to be secretive about their condition to change the culture in which they have grown up. Yet it is the actions of the adults in a family that most influence the actions of children. It is difficult to teach open and honest communication in this altered situation.

In addition to the issues surrounding disclosure of HIV status, there was frequently a reluctance to tell those children who were adopted about their adoptive status:

> One adoptive mother, the biological aunt, had not told her 14-year-old of his HIV status. The medical team was working with her to disclose this information, both because the teen was at an age where sexual activity was on his agenda and because he wanted to get working papers for which he needed his birth certificate. The aunt's reluctance to tell her son his HIV status was due to the fact he was old enough to figure out that if he was HIV-positive and she was not, then she was not his biological mother. This is a secret she had kept for 14 years and it was clear that she did not want to reveal it now.

Family illness

Life-threatening illnesses in childhood are seen as family illnesses as everyone in the family is affected when children are ill. HIV is unique both because, although not an illness as such, everyone is impacted by the condition and because more than one person in the family has it. Sometimes, every member of the nuclear family is HIV-positive. As a result, there are 'emotional' connections to the condition for everyone and every family member plays a role. Given the nature of HIV, each of these relationships can influence the sexual development of the child or young person.

Are grandmothers whose own children have died from HIV, or lost custody of their children because they were too ill or had too many social problems, more liberal with their grandchildren than they were with their own children – or more demanding? There are some grandmothers living for the care of their non-infected HIV grandchildren. Grandparents may feel as if they failed with their children and are being given a second chance by raising their grandchildren. However, taking care of your grandchild when your own adult child is incapable or too ill (or deceased) to care for their child can also be daunting. For families in which issues of substance abuse were the precursors to the HIV, grandmothers taking on the care of their grandchildren have shown tremendous resilience in their desire and efforts to have something good come of a difficult situation. Kinship care has been a remarkable response to family preservation and resilience (Scannapieco and Jackson 1996) in the AIDS epidemic.

Sibling issues are also complicated in families affected by HIV. There may be variability in the number of siblings infected, but all are affected. Younger siblings may rely on older siblings for guidance in their choices about sexual relations. If encouraged to talk about these issues, siblings can be a great support to one another.

Many unanswered questions

In the process of understanding the development of sexuality and intimacy in relationships for HIV-positive children, many areas worthy of assessment and exploration emerge. Among the questions for enquiry are:

1. Do you think about sexual behaviour differently if you grow up knowing that your parent is HIV-positive?

2. What are children's feelings for parents from whom they contracted the condition?

3. Do you think about sexuality differently if you grow up HIV-positive?

4. Is it influenced by the age at which you find yourself to be HIV-positive?

5. Does knowledge of advanced illness or mortality of a parent as the result of a sexually transmitted disease make you more aware of both your mortality and your sexuality, regardless of whether or not you are HIV-positive?

6. If you are HIV-positive, how do these factors influence your choices about relationships, partner notification, becoming a parent and so on?

7. Does the route of transmission of your parent's HIV status influence your behaviour?

8. What determines whether a child or young person who is HIV-positive develops positive or negative coping styles with regard to their own health?

9. Does the age that you learn that you are HIV-positive impact on your coping?

10. How is it that one child at ten can be very mature whereas another child of a similar age can be quite immature?

11. What defines maturity in the lives of children who have been brought up in a world of loss, secrecy and untruths?

12. Is the expectation for HIV-positive teens to use 'mature' judgment, and to be honest and open with those around them, in the interest of society when they may very well come from a family with a long history of hidden communication?

13. What are appropriate expectations for this cohort of children ageing into adolescence and young adulthood?

Sexual acting out can be an emotional response in many different situations – including to one's own feelings regarding transmission of HIV, the burden of illness, anger or isolation. To what degree are these issues open for discussion within families and with professionals?

Both mental health and medical providers are challenged by the lack of open communication among family members and with professional staff. There are situations when the health or social work professional knows that the child or young person is sexually active when the caregiver has no idea and insists that the child not be disclosed to. This brings ethical challenges to the forefront for the provider. What are the rights of the child or young person versus the family who care for them? And how do you respect the needs of both without disclosing confidential information about one to the other? What is the obligation to society?

Parental illness as a factor

Knowing of the advanced illness or mortality of a parent has a dramatic effect on the developing child. One study examined adolescent adjustment before and after an HIV-related parental death (Rotheram-Borus *et al.* 2005). Sexual risk behaviours increased after death and were sustained over the subsequent year and beyond. While the authors attribute this to adolescent developmental intimacy, it also may reflect the teens' need to 'connect' in the face of such a loss and combat ongoing feelings of isolation and depression.

In cases where the parent is alive, there is often an enormous sense of guilt regarding transmission to the child and a strong need to protect the child from further harm:

> I don't want to talk with her about [sex] because I don't want to give her any ideas. I don't want her making the same mistakes I did. (Parent of child at Mount Sinai Hospital)

The worry is both about children having sex and, as a result, putting others at risk. However, not talking about it does not prevent the child or young person from having sex. Additionally, many parents of HIV-positive children do not want to talk about sex or HIV with other people in case the dialogue forces other disclosures about the parent's past. It:

> ...opens a huge can of worms – I'm not ready to go there yet. I don't want her knowing what I did. (Parent of child at Mount Sinai Hospital)

> An HIV-positive teenager who was pregnant excitedly told her mother. Her mother said that, if she kept the child, she would kick her out of the house. The teen was forced to have an abortion. This is a situation in which the mother is also HIV-positive. The mother could not bear the thought of her own daughter having to live with the same guilt that she did. This places the child at emotional risk. How can she believe that her mother cares for her [as an HIV-positive teenager] when she demanded she abort a child because the child might be HIV-positive?

HIV-positive children and the experience of pregnancy

Pregnancy and the choices that people make in life about pregnancy can be complicated. In the case of children and young people who are HIV-positive, the choices about having a child may be conscious or unconscious, spoken or unspoken. There is research that suggests that those who lack emotional support and stability look to early sex and motherhood to provide closeness (Horwitz *et al.* 1991; Musick 1993). It has also been suggested that those with limited life options and choices are more likely to become pregnant (Coley and Chase-Lansdale 1998).

> In one situation there was a teenager who was quite aware that she was gravely ill. She wanted to do everything in a short time frame. For her, getting pregnant was a way of strengthening the connection to her boyfriend. She had a child about a year and a half before she died. The baby was not infected.

Among the psychodynamics of teens having children is the perception that they may feel the need (conscious or unconscious) to leave a legacy, to live on in a healthy, HIV-negative child. For others who have lost family members to AIDS, the desire to have a baby can be seen as a way to begin to fill the void, to begin to have their family:

> One teen talked about her sense of isolation. She had lost her mother, father, sister and grandmother to AIDS. She wanted to have a child to create a family as she had no remaining relatives.

> In another situation the teen's HIV was behaviourally acquired but her mother was also HIV-positive. The role for unconscious motivation behind not protecting oneself during sexual activity when one is aware of HIV and lives in a home with someone who is HIV-positive must be thought about. This mother had a younger HIV-infected child. This teen had a healthy, HIV-negative child and was able to give her mother the gift of a 'healthy child' to live in her household.

The dynamics in HIV-positive families influence not only the HIV-positive youth's approach to sex but also other components of life. HIV-positive children who are perinatally infected may have apprehensions about having a child because they understand the experience of being born affected. On the one hand, there are the fantasies of having a child who would be just like you and whose life would emulate your own. On the other, there is the fear of having a child who will be HIV-positive as you have been and who will have to live with the associated demands.

In some ways, having a HIV-negative child in a family living with HIV can symbolize the 'undoing' of the illness in a way that no one who is HIV-positive can do, even by living longer on a lifetime of medications. Many teens and young adults want to be giving to their mothers. As they deal with issues of their own condition and feelings of inadequacy at being HIV-positive (and anger at the parent for transmission), they seek alternatives that allow them to feel they are 'escaping' or leaving it behind. There is a belief that they can in fact move away from HIV by having a healthy child. Currently perinatal transmission has been on the decline and nearly eliminated in the United States in those situations in which mothers have access to health care and the ability to adhere to retroviral regimens:

> In another situation a young adult, in college and doing well, was someone no one thought would get pregnant but did. She saw herself as 'sick' and not like everyone else. For her, the idea of having a baby who was not sick made her feel more normal and less at the mercy of HIV.

> One teen described sex as the one area in her life where she was 'just like everyone else'. When her partners were unaware of her status and wanted to engage her in sex, she felt desirable. HIV made her feel 'ugly' and 'dirty'; when she was sexually attractive to another person those bad feelings went away.

Implications for HIV-positive children and young people

To be a teenager and to have a sexually transmitted disease that was not acquired through sexual transmission opens up a whole new arena for observation. The emotional implications have not been studied.

When you are born HIV-positive, there is a feeling of having no control over your life. Nothing you did got you to be HIV-positive and nothing you can do can get you to be HIV-negative. Disclosing one's HIV status places a great strain on relationships, meaning there is no such thing as a casual relationship. Knowing one is HIV-positive and choosing not to disclose places an even greater emotional pressure (even if being responsible and careful) on the youth who is HIV-positive. Carrying the secret can be untenable. Knowing one is HIV-positive and not using protection imposes great risk, presents an emotional burden to carry and imposes potential harm on someone else. However, feelings of immortality, seemingly counter-intuitive to

HIV-positive youth who have seen family members die from HIV, still prevail. Even HIV-positive youngsters can have the belief that bad things will not happen to them.

There are many unanswered questions and ethical issues for practitioners to consider. It is through clinical work with individuals that some understanding of these issues is emerging. In a group of six mental health professionals working with perinatally infected children and young people in New York City particular concerns emerged about:

- perinatally infected adolescents becoming sexually active before and after knowing their HIV status

- sexually active adolescents' willingness (or lack thereof) to disclose to sexual partners

- family members' lack of acceptance or denial that their child is sexually active coupled with medical providers' lack of acceptance or denial of the sexual activity

- learned powerlessness on the part of children, young people and families who feel they have succumbed to HIV.

We came up with the following initial guidelines for practitioners:

- Allow children and young people of all ages the opportunity for expression.

- Talk with HIV-positive youth about sex and about responsibility.

- Expect that in any situation there may be more complicated issues because of the nature of HIV and its transmission.

- Begin a dialogue about the underlying issues that many of these youth face.

- Create a network of HIV-positive youth to help one another.

- Acknowledge the challenges imposed by living with HIV and being in an HIV-positive family.

- Be a leader in raising difficult issues so teens know that there is a resource for them.

- Provide the opportunity for youth to make safe and responsible choices, even at a developmental stage, which may contradict the concept of 'safe and responsible'.

Conclusion

Each of the factors related to the social climate into which this population was born, the social climate in which they are living and each individual's family story affect the ways in which children, teens and young adults perinatally infected with HIV see themselves, their sexuality and their mortality.

If no one has ever travelled on this road before you, and you are caught in the context of a health condition in which 'secrecy' has been the norm, it is difficult to identify role models who can help guide the way. Within this population of those emerging into adulthood is the legacy of the people in their lives who have died of AIDS. Growing up HIV-positive can destroy some families and have a significant impact on others. Sex can become a way for children, teens and young adults who may feel 'disenfranchised' or disconnected from their peers to feel connected. Given the nature of transmission of HIV and the vulnerability of these children and young people because of their many losses, the burdens they carry and the chronic nature of their illness, issues of sexuality, childbearing and transmission of HIV are central. Increasingly, health and social work professionals must feel comfortable finding ways to bring these issues into the dialogue in the interest of helping this cohort in what has otherwise been uncharted territory.

14

Young Adult Cancer Survivors
Shaken Up, Getting Back, Moving On

Brad Zebrack

Introduction

> Dr Chatham called last night with the results of your biopsy, Brad. He'd like for you to check into the hospital tomorrow morning to run some additional tests. The preliminary results show that you have Hodgkin's disease. It's a form of cancer, and you're going to have to put your life on hold for about a year while you undergo treatment.

Although the doctor said my chances for cure were high, I thought 'But it's still cancer!' and I wondered if I would become some sickly kind of guy for the rest of my life. Fortunately, I've been far from sickly. I am, and have been for almost 20 years, in full recovery. Since having cancer I have been hiking and backpacking and bicycling all over the United States. I went to graduate school and am now a Professor of Social Work at the University of Southern California where I am researching how cancer impacts the lives of patients and their families. Most notably, three years ago I achieved a milestone that I thought for a long time would never happen due to the effects of chemotherapy on my fertility. I became a father.

Life tasks and challenges in adolescent and young adult cancer survivors

The end of cancer treatment, returning to school or work, leaving home, dating, starting a family and/or a career and establishing regular and appropriate health care are all important stages of young adult cancer survivors' lives. These life stages carry with them the potential for new understandings of cancer's impact, new worries or concerns, and new challenges to physical health and abilities. It may be that at certain life transitions some survivors find their worries realized, find it difficult to obtain insurance or employment, recognize the limitations of their mental abilities or social skills, or understand the meaning and realities of chemotherapy's effect on fertility (Dolgin *et al.* 1999; Roberts *et al.* 1997). These life stages also may be times when the cancer experience becomes a personal resource that motivates survivors to help others, or instils in them an inner sense of confidence, purpose and knowledge about what is important in life (Chesler, Weigers and Lawther 1992).

Coping with cancer throughout survivorship requires an individual to continuously appraise cancer's threat and potential for change as it appears and re-appears in different forms at various times throughout the remainder of life (for example, as threat to reproduction; as discrimination when seeking insurance or employment; when starting a family; when certain environmental stimuli remind the survivor of his/her experience; when other friends or family members are diagnosed with cancer; if or when a recurrence or second cancer is diagnosed). Cancer survivors confront, on various occasions, reminders of their cancer and thus have multiple opportunities to experience either positive or negative feelings associated with the illness. They see television programmes and commercials with cancer-related themes, receive announcements regarding support groups, picnics and celebrations, hear through various media outlets about meetings with other cancer survivors and learn of family members, friends or acquaintances diagnosed with cancer. All these messages may evoke, or help survivors express and experience, a new or renewed sense of self. They may cause them to perceive, perhaps for the very first time, strong feelings related to having had cancer as a child or teenager.

Theories of psychological maturation and growth identify life tasks that older adolescents and young adults face, such as establishing intimate relationships, continuing education, making career and work choices, establishing independent living and planning a family (Gould 1972; Levinson and Gooden 1985). These issues, challenging in the best of circumstances, are often compounded and complicated by a cancer diagnosis, its treatment and subsequent long-term physical and psycho-social effects. Furthermore, self-concept is a key determinant of the impact of major life changes, for valued aspects of the self (i.e. attitudes, beliefs and values) regulate the meaning, importance and thus the impact of various life experiences on individuals (Pearlin 1989). Empirical findings in the quality of life literature imply that positive psycho-social adjustment for some cancer survivors is associated with an ability to integrate the experience into one's self-concept by deriving meaning from the cancer experience, creating changes in life priorities or accepting one's mortality (Gray *et al.* 1992a; Taylor 1993).

Social activity and relationships

Young adulthood is a time of increased vulnerability to stress and social pressures and presents cancer survivors with major developmental challenges above and beyond those faced by other young people (Hobbie *et al.* 2000). For example, negotiating interpersonal relationships (including intimacy and forming families), as well as educational and employment decisions and achievements, often requires a focus, perhaps for the first time, on the medical, social, cognitive or psychological effects of cancer treatment. It is not uncommon for adolescents and young adults with cancer to experience changes in friendships and perhaps a sense of isolation from friends due to lengthy time away from home, school or work for treatments; many friendships may fall by the wayside over time (Schultz Adams 2003). Adolescents and young adults with cancer may become isolated from friends who they feel may no longer be able to relate to their life situation. These young patients and survivors report that their friends get uncomfortable continuously talking with them about cancer and as a result they begin to feel 'different' and perhaps apprehensive about forming new friendships (Chesler *et al.* 1992). Consequently, these young people often form new friendship circles, especially as a function of increased maturity and letting go of immature friends. For some, particularly those with brain tumours, the consequences of cancer include being fatigued, perceived by peers as sick, often absent from school and selected less often than healthy peers as a best friend, thereby resulting in social isolation (Vanatta *et al.* 1998).

While childhood cancer survivors often describe improvements in relationships with friends and family, they also indicate greater disappointment in those relationships when compared with controls (Gray *et al.* 1992b). Gray *et al.* suggest that this disappointment is a result of having higher expectations. Thus, it would be incorrect to assume that reported improvements in social relationships are necessarily a positive outcome. Indeed, Chesler and Barbarin (1984) noted that existing social networks may fail to provide the type or kind of support that long-term survivors seek or may even cause additional stress.

Self-concept, body image, sexual identity

Cancer has the potential to influence development of self-concept, a key task, among young people (Rowland 1990). Alterations in physical appearance, including weight changes, hair loss, amputations, placement of catheters to facilitate treatment administration, scars and alterations in skin colouration and texture, not only make children and teens feel different from peers but also may represent frightening changes in the body with an adverse impact on self-esteem. Fears that the body will never return to its original appearance, of not being recognized by others or of being mistaken for an individual of the opposite sex, often lead to shame, social isolation, and regressive behaviours (Die-Trill and Stuber 1998). These sometimes sudden alterations in body image are often perceived by patients as a threat to their well-being, causing anxiety. Also, self-image and life outlook appear to be worse among survivors who perceive treatment-related physical limitation as being moderate to severe when compared with survivors who perceive late effects as being only mildly or not at all limiting (Zebrack and Chesler 2001). It is notable that the *perception* of limitation and not an actual physical or visible 'disability' appears related to self-image and life outlook. For example, respondents who indicated mild or no limitations included individuals with amputations or other noticeable effects of treatment (i.e. scars), suggesting that some survivors with physical or visible effects of cancer did not necessarily see themselves as having limitations.

Chemotherapy and radiation treatments sometimes make patients feel as if their bodies are not their own. Their well-remembered physical responses often are thrown out of kilter by the mood-changing and physique-altering effects of drugs. Changes in body image stem from both the physical effects of treatment and the wrenching feeling that there is an internal battle going on between good cells and bad cells (Chesler and Barbarin 1987). Some investigators have noted that for adolescents, changes in appearance (i.e. hair loss, weight gain) are even more troublesome than the pain of treatments (Orr, Hoffmans and Bennetts 1984).

Many adolescents report that the treatment is worse than the disease (Ross and Scarvalone 1982) and that the bodily changes that accompany chemotherapy and radiation make it more difficult to develop a positive body image (Zeltzer 1993). The effect on physical appearance is especially disruptive for females (Zeltzer *et al.* 1980). Pendley, Dahlquist and Dreyer (1997) examined body image in adolescents who completed treatment and found that adolescents who had been off treatment longer reported more negative body image perceptions and that childhood cancer survivors may not recognize body image concerns until several years after treatment ends. Whether based on reality or not, persistent negative perceptions may result in a loss of sex appeal and virility or a distorted body image producing feelings of inferiority, low self-esteem and incompetence (Zeltzer 1993).

A special consideration related to self-image is the subject of sexual identity. It is during adolescence that individuals come to realize that they are sexual beings; adolescents begin to develop sexual identities and conceptualize their reproductive capacity. Adolescents display concern about attractiveness to peers and many begin to explore intimate relationships. It is not surprising, then, that cancer and associated treatments and side-effects would impact on their burgeoning sexuality. In a self-report survey assessing sexual attitudes and experiences of 30 adolescent and young adult survivors and 50 healthy age-matched controls, Puukko and colleagues (1997) reported that survivors differed significantly from controls with regard to their inner sense of sexuality, with images of sexuality being more restrictive and attitudes being more negative, although age at initiation of dating and sexual activity, frequency of sexual intercourse and opinions on sexual behaviour were similar in both groups. In comparing the sexual concerns of adolescent patients with those of a healthy comparison group, Chambas (1991) reported that adolescents with cancer commonly raised concerns about the impact of treatment, whereas healthy teens' concerns centred around physical appearance or puberty. While healthy adolescent girls expressed concerns about pregnancy (it could 'ruin my life') adolescent cancer patients were more concerned about the potential effects of treatment on their future ability to have children.

The comment from a childhood cancer survivor below exemplifies how young adult survivors' sense of self and 'feeling normal' may be associated with perceived peer expectations and uncertainty about whether or not they may be able to have children of their own:

> When they said I couldn't get pregnant I was very upset. I felt guilty, like it was something I wouldn't be able to do and everybody else could do it. All these teenagers were having children and not wanting them, and I wouldn't even have a choice... I wasn't exactly the cautious teenager. I just didn't think I could have children. We

didn't use a lot of protection, because I thought I couldn't... You just think that every woman should be able to have kids and that's the one thing you were made to do, is to have children. And when you're told that you may not, you don't even have the option of doing that, it's taken away from you, then you feel horrible, because you definitely want one when they say you can't have one... I thought I was just weird. I remember praying when I was 19 and saying, 'God, why can't I just be like all the other girls? Why can't I just have kids? Why can't I have that option, why can't you give me that option?' And no sooner did I say that, I had my son. I got pregnant a couple months later. It was weird, but I just wanted to be like them [other friends having babies], I wanted to be normal... Most girls they think they're gonna keep a man by getting pregnant. That's not why I was doing it. I was doing it because I wanted to have a baby. I wanted to see if I could have a baby. (Zebrack *et al.* 2004, pp.689–699)

Fertility

Prior to starting my own chemotherapy treatment, my doctor informed me that I most likely would become infertile from the drugs that would cure my cancer. Being so focused on living and (not) dying, I was not really thinking or worrying about having children later. However, my doctor suggested sperm-banking as the answer to my probable treatment-induced sterility.

Suggesting that sperm-banking is the answer to infertility is like saying that chemotherapy is the answer to cancer. There is an element of truth, but the reality is far more complex; there are no guarantees. Furthermore, this 'answer' pertains only to men. The options for women are far more complex and invasive and just as uncertain (see Chapters 5 and 6).

Most research on fertility and pregnancy outcomes after treatment has reported primarily on the risks for infertility in cancer survivors. Current knowledge regarding reproductive effects in young adult survivors of adult-onset and childhood cancer focuses primarily on treatment-related risk factors for infertility and other reproductive organ/gonadal effects, including early menopause (Byrne 1999a; Kwon and Case 2002). Fertility preservation and pregnancy outcomes, including effects of treatment on progeny of childhood survivors and risks for congenital defects and cancer, also have been evaluated (Aslam *et al.* 2000; Blatt 1999; Byrne 1999b). Some reports go as far as to mention artificial insemination, *in vitro* fertilization, or adoption as options for the future (Meirow 2000) but no studies report the extent to which cancer survivors utilize these services or their experiences with them.

Research indicates that adolescent and young adult cancer survivors worry about their ability to have children and/or the health of their off-spring (Langeveld et al. 2003; Schover et al. 1999; Weigers et al. 1998). Additional reports suggest infertility comes as a surprise and many young adult survivors do not recall being warned at the time of their treatment that they were risking their fertility (Schover 1999; Zebrack et al. 2004). Others studying cancer survivorship in young adults have indicated that concerns about raising children, when to share one's cancer history with a new part-ner and the impact of treatment on sexuality, intimacy and relationships are of the utmost importance (Roberts et al. 1997; Thaler-Demers 2001). Young adult survivors have expressed concerns about how and when to divulge the possibility of infertility with potential spouses or life partners; some express fears of being rejected as a result (Zebrack et al. 2004). The following comment from a young woman survivor of childhood cancer illustrates these fears:

> That was one of our big problems, because he wanted kids. I didn't know, maybe the chemo did something. He goes, 'Well, there's people that take chemo and have all kinds of kids.' [Pause] We're still friends now. And he just had a baby, and he had to come over here and tell me that he had a baby, like it was kind of throwing it in my face. (Zebrack et al. 2004, pp.689–699)

Many young adult survivors faced with the potential loss of having children experience assurances from well-meaning family, friends and health profes-sionals who say things like 'You can always adopt', or 'You know, they've made so many advances in technology these days...' These 'solutions', however, are neither adequate nor informative; they are simplistic and do not offer a realistic picture of what young adult survivors may experience when it comes time to think seriously about starting a family.

In addition to the physiological consequences described above, fertility issues have repercussions in other aspects of survivors' lives. With regard to attitudes about the importance of family, some survivors' responses reflect resilience and enhanced appreciation for life through being able to have a child after believing that doing so was impossible or unlikely. Their com-ments suggest that the experience of surviving cancer may enhance one's confidence and skill as a current or future parent (Schover et al. 1999). In contrast, a perceived loss of opportunity for parenthood in some cases may be devastating to self-esteem and potentially damaging to marital or other intimate relationships.

My path to parenthood

As adolescent and young adult cancer survivors age and mature, they appear to lack critical information necessary to make informed choices about family planning including regarding their cancer and its treatment; types and dosages of treatment; in some cases, even the type of cancer they had; and knowledge about potential long-term physical effects (Kadan-Lottick *et al.* 2002). Given that there is a general lack of knowledge about the anatomy and physiology of reproduction among adolescents in general and that this lack of knowledge is often accompanied by heightened curiosity about sexuality and experimentation with intimacy and sex (Heiney 1989), adolescent and young adult cancer survivors must cope with the impact of diagnosis and treatment as it may affect their sexual identity and sexual behaviour in ways unique and specific to cancer survivors (Zebrack *et al.* 2004).

Seven years after my own treatment I was finally ready to make a 'withdrawal' from the sperm bank. Only then did I begin to understand the lifelong implications of cancer treatment on my fertility, along with the complex processes involved in artificial insemination and technology-aided methods of conception.

Given that my wife and I were ready to have children we had to figure out what to do. We started low-tech and low cost with a procedure we sarcastically called the 'turkey-baster' method. After learning how to chart my wife's ovulation cycle and observing it for several months, we were ready to predict a window of ovulation with some certainty. At this point I went to the fertility centre to withdraw one vial of my cryogenically preserved sperm. At home I thawed it in warm water just as the lab technician described. Then, following directions, I used a syringe and plastic tube to inject reconstituted semen into my wife's cervix. We tried this procedure a couple of times with no luck.

Second, we identified two local fertility specialists, interviewed them and eventually prepared for a more invasive and expensive *in vitro* fertilization procedure. This involved injecting my wife with mood-altering hormones and fertility drugs over several months to prepare her body for egg retrieval and later implantation of a fertilized embryo. I recall feeling guilt about being the cancer survivor yet subjecting my wife to invasive and discomforting procedures, being angry at cancer, eight years after diagnosis and treatment, for subjecting both of us to these trying procedures. After expending two vials of sperm and $8000, the placement of a fertilized egg in her womb did not result in a successful pregnancy.

We discussed the option of not having children at all. We realized that electing childlessness was a viable option, a choice we could make. It meant that children would become part of our lives in different ways – through our brothers, sisters and friends. For five years this option offered a sense of freedom that some of our friends with children envied. However, I started to feel life had more to offer, so I brought up the subject of children again and suggested we look into adoption.

Adoption in the USA can come in many forms. There are closed adoptions brokered through attorneys and adoption agencies, both international and domestic and adoption through foster care. We chose 'open adoption', a procedure in which we developed and now maintain an ongoing relationship with our daughter's biological parents. Getting to this point, however, took almost two years and involved a series of bureaucratic and sometimes emotionally taxing steps.

We began our journey to parenthood by locating and enlisting with a state-sponsored adoption agency and attending a 'Pathways to Parenthood' adoption orientation class. Classes were followed by a series of state-required meetings with social workers, including visits to our home. Meanwhile, we created a 'parent profile' and 'birthmother letter' – two documents introducing us as potential parents for a child, which the agency would share with women who approached them about placing an unborn child for adoption. Eventually we received a call from our social worker telling us that a birthmother was interested in meeting us.

As we proceeded with meeting her we were uncertain how things would turn out, but if cancer taught me anything it is that life is full of uncertainty. While I have become comfortable with uncertainty, it is not always easy and can lead to disappointment, as it did in this first try at adoption. After three months of getting to know the woman who would bear us a child, she changed her mind when the baby was born and decided to keep her child (which was well within her rights). We were emotionally devastated and endured days dealing with wavering and alternating feelings of disappointment, anger, compassion and eventually determination to have a child of our own.

After a period of comforting and renewing our intention, we reinitiated our efforts and were soon selected by a young couple. The experience was remarkably different from the first attempt but still fraught with uncertainty at times. Over a two-and-a-half-month period we spent time with the birthparents, which included buying maternity clothes, walking on the beach, going together for pre-natal doctors' visits and attended birthing classes. Ultimately, we were present at the birth of our daughter Sierra Grace.

Implications for follow-up and long-term care

Today, not enough is known about the challenges facing adolescents and young adults with a history of childhood cancer, or about the strategies they may use to effectively address them, or about the programmes and interventions that may effectively increase knowledge about cancer and its treatment, empowerment, self-confidence and coping. This is in part due to the fact that follow-up care for young adult survivors of paediatric and adult-onset cancers is not consistently provided in the same setting in which they receive their cancer treatment. Oeffinger *et al.* (1998) report that 'few programs focus on the long-term health care needs of adult survivors of childhood cancer. The majority of existing programs are in pediatric institutions, without significant input from adult-oriented, generalist health care providers' (p.2864). Oncology professionals must consider where and when as well as how best to deliver interventions that will meet the needs of a young, developing and geographically mobile population. We need to proactively empower and prepare survivors during their treatment through the teaching of advocacy skills and we may need to bring follow-up intervention to the client, or at least provide it in settings appropriate and conducive to their needs.

Harvey *et al.* (1999) suggest that comprehensive and quality follow-up for long-term cancer survivors should include education in previous diagnosis, treatment and potential late effects, with an emphasis on wellness, health maintenance and health promotion. Fertility assessment, including evaluation of survivors' knowledge about their own reproductive capacity, and counselling should become part of that comprehensive follow-up. Young adult survivors, as well as the health and welfare professionals who care for them, may benefit from timely information and health education regarding present and future fertility, options for having a family, sexual behaviour and risks for adverse outcomes such as unplanned pregnancy or exposure to sexually transmitted diseases (STDs).

As these young people age, the transition from being patients to off-treatment survivors and the taking on of new and additional responsibilities as they establish independence mean they will be faced with making their own life decisions. An important issue for adolescent and young adults is the decision of if, when and how to share information about cancer with their peers. An even more delicate issue is what and how much to say about their illness to new acquaintances and particularly to those with whom a long-term intimate relationship may be possible. Faced with the potential for varied reactions, young people with cancer may lose confidence because of their uncertainty about whether and how they will be accepted. When loss of opportunities for social interaction with peers is severe, it is experienced as a major deprivation that multiplies other stresses of the illness. When positive interaction with peers occurs, it helps ease such stresses and renews young people's adaptive capacities. Given that peer socialization and relationships are of great importance and concern to this young population, those who promote an advocacy framework for support are faced with the challenge of developing a skill set that will help survivors deal with stigmatization by peers and maintain friendships/relationships.

Peer support and support groups

As an educator and patient advocate with over 20 years of experience with environmental education programmes, summer camps and oncology camps for children, I have witnessed the personal growth and development that occurs in young people who participate in peer support programmes. However, older adolescents and young adult cancer survivors are rarely afforded these opportunities. For young adults diagnosed with cancer and faced with an extraordinary situation that 'rocks their world', peer support programmes can offer an environment of safety and encouragement that is not otherwise available to them.

Roberts *et al.* (1997) report results of a support group intervention designed to facilitate adjustment in young adults with cancer. Improvements in psychological well-being were observed. The group was facilitated by two young adults, one of each gender. Topics covered included anxiety about health and physical well-being, worries about fertility and raising children, relationship problems, financial concerns and body image. The authors noted that the group quickly developed cohesion and they suggested that the quickness and ease with which this happened was demonstrative of the participants' need and desire for support. Indeed, more than half of a sample of 303 survivors aged 14–29 indicated a need or desire to meet other adolescent or young adult survivors (Zebrack and Chesler 2000).

Thus, participation in oncology camps, outdoor adventure programmes, cancer survivor day picnics and family retreats offers opportunities for life experiences that promote successful achievement of age-appropriate developmental tasks. For instance, a wilderness adventure programme provides adolescents undergoing therapy with extraordinary experiences that boost self-image and facilitate coping skills (Stevens *et al.* 2004). An eight-day adventure trip for 17 young adult survivors of childhood cancer provided an opportunity for physical challenges and resulted in reports of improvements in self-confidence, independence and social contacts (Elad *et al.* 2003). These participants also indicated a preference for confronting the impact of cancer in their lives through the use of humour, religious beliefs, cognitive reframing and imagination. Opportunities for peer involvement provide young survivors with a chance to address areas of mutual concern, such as coping with uncertainty, social exclusion, separation from parents, body image, intimacy, sexuality and fertility, with others whom they can observe as sharing similar experiences.

Conclusion

Cancer survivors and health and welfare professionals can benefit from information derived from research on infertility risks and associated psychological and behavioural outcomes, as well as from current information on available alternatives for having children, genetic risks, risks for unplanned pregnancy and risks for exposure to STDs. Research also suggests that professionals working in the health care arena may benefit from information and training on how and when to broach fertility issues with their patients (Cartwright-Alcarese 1995; Koeppel 1995). Several relatively new support agencies in the USA, Fertile Hope (www.fertilehope.org), the Ulman Family Fund for Young Adults (www.ulmanfund.org), Planet Cancer (www.planetcancer.org) and the Lance Armstrong Foundation (www.laf.org), are addressing specific psycho-social needs of young adult cancer survivors and providing accurate and appropriate knowledge regarding fertility options, as well as much needed emotional support.

As for me, I am involved in raising a child at a time when many of my same-aged friends, relatives and colleagues are seeing their children off to high school and college. It is not the first time I have had to deal with life challenges or opportunities occurring out of what might be considered a normal timeline for people my age, but it is something with which I am comfortable. How could I not be, when there is nothing better than coming home from work and having my two-year-old daughter greet me and say, 'Missed you Dada.'

15.

Becoming a Parent – the Transition to Parenthood Where There is Pre-existing Fertility Impairment

Mary Self[1]

Introduction

Two decades ago, as an adolescent, I was treated for bone cancer with an amputation of my leg and chemotherapy. At the time it was unthinkable that professionals would consider the problems of teenagers, having survived cancer, then going on to make decisions involving parenthood. Not only was the prognosis for such patients gloomy, but long-term effects of cancer treatments on fertility were unknown.

With the greatly improved outlook for teen-cancer-survivors, advances in assisted reproduction techniques and a shifting emphasis towards the implications of long-term survival, attention is now being drawn to the impact of diagnosis and treatment on the desire and ability to become a parent. Clinicians are considering the psycho-social challenges facing teenagers with impaired fertility as they graduate into the societal roles accompanying adulthood.

I write this chapter from several perspectives. First, as a teen-cancer-survivor who has contemplated the sadness of infertility. Second, I write as a psychiatrist with an interest in the psycho-social implications of cancer diagnosis and subsequent treatment. Finally, I write as a mother discovering that long-term survival encompasses helping my two young children to have a healthy understanding of cancer.

I shall address this subject both from an experiential and a research-based approach. Excellent research exists documenting the potential of treatment modalities to cause physical complications such as infertility, spontaneous abortion, congenital anomalies and cancer in survivors' offspring. However, very little evidence exists enabling us to understand the psychological conflicts caused by long-term insults to reproductive life. Answers are beginning to emerge but remain sparse and inconclusive.

I have asked many questions on my journey of survival. I have discovered many answers are far from clear. The fearful uncertainty of 'Will I live?' has faded with each clear check-up, only for a new question to take its place. 'Can I have children?' became uppermost in my mind as I realized I had a future. This question itself led to many more on the path of survivorship and the hope of parenthood.

Permit me in this chapter to share some of my questions and experiences in the hope they may broaden our understanding and inspire further research.

Question one: am I fertile?

17 years old: a week before starting chemotherapy

> Today I asked my consultant the question that has been really worrying me. I accept I had to lose my leg and I have cancer. Now I am really worried whether I can have children. I asked two doctors already and they said probably chemo will make me infertile but to ask the consultant oncologist because she is the expert. So I plucked up courage to ask her, 'Will I be able to have children?' First I was not sure if she had heard me because she carried on looking at the notes. Then she looked at me as if I had grown two heads and then she said, 'Let's get you through this first shall we?' I don't think anyone here realizes just how important it is to me. I love kids and having them means everything to me, even more than being a doctor. If I can't have any what's the point of being alive? But whenever I mention it everybody goes quiet on me. And sitting here not knowing and not being given any answers is worse than knowing the truth. So I asked another doctor, the senior registrar who is next most important. He said, 'No, you won't be able to have any.' Then he walked off and now I have this dark, cold emptiness

inside me because something else really important has been taken away from me.

For cancer survivors diagnosed in childhood, adolescence or young adult life, the impact of various cancer treatments on subsequent fertility is a vital issue. Not only does the possibility of fertility impairment produce more uncertainty for the individual but it also marks them out as different from their peer group. It represents a significant limitation in achieving future life goals and a loss of normal functioning and health. All these factors produce additional marked psychological stress for the young person in a situation that is already deeply traumatic.

Despite widespread acceptance of the sadness caused by infertility, research shows that communication in this area is neglected. A study by Schover *et al.* in 1999 showed that 57 per cent of young survivors receiving cancer treatment cannot recall ever discussing the possibility of infertility with their specialists even though half of the original study sample viewed themselves as having impaired fertility (Schover *et al.* 1999). Only 26 per cent of childless male survivors banked sperm before treatment, a low figure given that the technique of *in vitro* fertilization with intracytoplasmic sperm injection (IVF-ICSI) is now a well-established successful technique (Schover 1999).

Many difficulties exist surrounding discussion of potential infertility at the time of initial diagnosis and treatment. A young patient must assimilate many painful truths. The oncologist must breach sensitive topics: the loss of being able to have children, the need to explain masturbation to provide sperm samples and, of course, the likelihood of a youngster reaching child-bearing age. A teenager may not see future parenthood as relevant to them, especially in a time of illness, and may not completely remember the mass of highly distressing information. Parents try to protect a sick child from further distressing news and fear that a young person will refuse treatment if fully aware of all the side-effects. Many forms of cancer in younger patients are highly aggressive and treatment delay may be undesirable.

There is evidence to suggest that men who reject the option of sperm banking and remain childless later regret their decision (Cella and Najavits 1986). Infertility represents a major loss event and is emotionally painful, predisposing to depression in later years (Parkes and Markus 1998). This grief may be hidden and unacknowledged, representing a loss of potential rather than existing children. We do not know if infertility following cancer treatment is more traumatic than that of isolated infertility. It may be that cancer survivors see infertility as 'the sting in the tail' adding yet more sorrow to a painful situation. Conversely, a survivor may feel so relieved to be alive that the loss of fertility pales by comparison. Do survivors deny their true feelings concerning infertility out of a sense of guilt: 'I should just be grateful to be alive when others did not make it'? Or do they value life so highly after a close brush with death that creating a family seems more important? As yet, research has not provided full answers. Adjustment to impaired fertility is a dynamic process, evolving and changing over the years. Each survivor's attitudes will reflect individual personalities and ambitions, previous experiences and choices made in the context of illness.

Adolescents need to develop culturally appropriate levels of autonomy and independence. For the sick teenager, these important tasks are threatened and maintaining a feeling of control is crucial. Any loss of control will be overwhelmingly stressful. Therefore, honest, empathic communication concerning the likelihood of infertility and fertility-sparing options can help reduce subsequent distress. Access to fertility medical counselling at diagnosis, and throughout long-term follow-up, empowers young adults with accurate and up-to-date information. It also provides opportunities for research into the needs, anxieties, attitudes and psychological outcomes of those with fertility impairment.

Original fears that cancer treatments would produce a high rate of infertility have not been realized, being mostly restricted to alkylating agents and high doses of gonadally targeted radiotherapy. Without the facts acquired by sensitive fertility medical counselling, many young adults may be needlessly worrying. Long-term follow-up provides an opportunity to inform and reassure patients as they grow up and prognosis improves. Very often though, follow-up clinics are busy and access to relevant expertise may not be available. The follow-up process, by adopting a multi-disciplinary approach, must address the fears of young adults as they move from worrying about survival to contemplating a future. Survivors' interests extend beyond five-year-survival statistics to the practicalities of achieving life goals such as employment, marriage and having a family. Oncologists can greatly support a survivor in these tasks by liaising with appropriate specialities.

22 years old: a month before getting engaged

Today I asked my consultant again about having children. I told him I was getting married so I needed information. Today is my five-year check-up and he said it looks like I am going to be in the clear from secondaries, which is fantastic – but I want to get on with life now and do what all my friends are doing: getting jobs, marrying and thinking about babies. I just got the feeling my oncologist found my questions about babies embarrassing and he was pretty vague, saying there was not much research so they didn't really know but maybe not to get my hopes up because my fertility was bound to be *'impaired'*. I knew he had loads of patients to see and he seemed a bit reluctant to talk about it so I left feeling as if there is still this big question mark over my future. Maybe Richard won't want to get married if we can't have kids. Maybe we won't be able to cope with having a big hole in our life together where our kids should be. It just doesn't seem fair that cancer has taken my fertility away as well as my leg.

For those who discover that they have impaired fertility, a variety of assisted reproduction options exist, such as sperm banking and IVF-ICSI. Other techniques such as ovarian cryopreservation are in their experimental infancy. Options such as donor insemination, egg donation, surrogacy and adoption may be available to infertile couples. We do not yet know the emotional hurdles these procedures may present for the cancer survivor. Does the need for further medical intervention produce more distress and anxiety for a person who has undergone repeated hospitalizations in the past, or are survivors made more resilient by previous unpleasant treatment? Do adoption agencies, donors and surrogates view cancer survivors as potential parents or do they take a negative view of a past history of malignancy? We simply do not know, as few survivors have faced such situations. However, with improved survival, the number of young adults seeking answers to these questions will increase.

And what of those young adults who, having been warned of infertility, discover the return of reproductive ability? Is the news greeted with joy or is there a degree of mistrust towards oncologists? Without doubt, the return of fertility produces a whole new series of challenges and questions.

Question two: will cancer affect my pregnancy?

27 years old: ten weeks pregnant

> Now that I am pregnant with this precious child I have begun to worry so much about Baby's health. I never expected this and I am scared now in case something bad happens. Maybe Baby will be damaged by the chemotherapy. It destroyed my eggs all those years ago so what about the ones left behind? Chemotherapy was so toxic it made my hair fall out. So maybe my eggs could have been poisoned too. Maybe I'll give birth to a freak. I keep getting these frightening dreams that when Baby is born he has one big cyclops eye in the middle of a grotesquely deformed head. I told my obstetrician about having methotrexate and vincristine chemotherapy but he said he didn't know much about them; not exactly reassuring. I can't go back to the oncologists and ask them either, because I haven't been to my check-ups for ages and they stopped sending me appointments. I don't know where to go for answers so I'm just worrying and waiting to see if Baby is healthy.

The vast majority of mothers-to-be worry about the health of their unborn child. Cancer survivors have additional reasons to be concerned. Radiotherapy and chemotherapy were shown to be mutagenic agents in animal studies, but, until recent years, the potential for preconception treatment to cause mutagenic damage to human germ cells was unknown (Li *et al.* 1979). Several large studies looking at survivor pregnancy outcomes occurring years after treatment have been published within the last few years and are reassuring in this regard (Blatt 1999; Li *et al.* 1979). These studies have concluded that no adverse outcomes, in terms of excess congenital malformations, have been identified with most chemotherapeutic agents and the associated risk is very small.

Yet, even well-informed survivors do not appear to be aware of the reassuring nature of this evidence. One study showed that 18 per cent of fertile survivors underwent voluntary sterilization procedures, with almost half of the women stating that fear of pregnancy after cancer treatment was a major factor in their decision (Schover *et al.* 1999). Long-term follow-up clinics should ideally provide a forum for gathering and sharing information. However, this can present problems over the years with survivors lost to follow-up for a number of reasons. Follow-up may be seen as less relevant as disease-free time increases. The follow-up clinic tends to be conducted by junior doctors unaware of current research in this area and clinicians change over the years, leading to inconsistency in information-giving. Survivors graduate from paediatric and adolescent services to adult services and move geographically. As a result, access to information may be inadequate and communication of the facts sporadic. The priorities of clinician and survivor are inherently different: those of the clinician often being length of life, while the quality of that life is a survivor's priority. Once well, a young adult survivor may simply tire of being a 'patient' and default from follow-up, thereby losing the opportunity to obtain help, support and information in later years. Clinicians need to look at why survivors do not receive potentially reassuring news that can make such a difference to quality of life.

On the other hand, there is little evidence to suggest that survivors worry about more relevant issues such as increased risk of miscarriage, premature birth and having low birthweight babies (Critchley *et al.* 1992). Evidence shows that all these fears are justified after some chemotherapy regimes and particularly after pelvic irradiation. Again, survivors do not appear to be getting a clear picture and we must ask why. There may be scope for oncologists to liaise with obstetric colleagues in developing education and research initiatives. Informing survivors and professionals from overlapping disciplines could help to raise awareness as well as anticipating and preventing perinatal problems.

32 years old: ten weeks into my fourth pregnancy

I am ten weeks pregnant and I can't cope with another miscarriage and losing another embryonic life. The first miscarriage wasn't too bad – I lost the baby early on, about six weeks. It would have been difficult to cope with a toddler and a newborn. But it did cross my mind that maybe the chemotherapy might have been responsible. I didn't even go to the doctor at the time – just got on with recovering and forgetting how it felt to flush all those early baby hopes down the toilet. But the second time was horrendous; 16 weeks pregnant and I knew my baby. I'd seen her tiny form and felt her move inside me. I loved her and wanted her. I had so many dreams and then one day she was gone, with nothing to hold on to apart from my scan pictures. And I felt so bereft. I could not go through that again. I blame the chemotherapy now. Nobody told me it would do this but it cannot just be down to coincidence. If it hadn't been for those drugs my baby – even my babies – would still be alive. So this time I am playing it very cautiously; I booked under a Fetal Medicine

Specialist and told him all about my fears. He has been really supportive, explaining the research and scanning me every week or two in clinic to check on Baby's health. When I see the heartbeat I silently rejoice that this time the cancer and all that toxic poison has not got the better of us because my baby is alive and well.

Cancer may present in a young adult who has already borne children. Anxiety about infertility occurs in these survivors also (Schover 1999; Schover et al. 1999) as the choice to have more children is removed. Professionals, who may perceive the patient to be fortunate in having at least one child, can overlook this. However, the loss of building a bigger family having known the joy of parenthood can still be significant. There may be worries about an existing offspring growing up as an only child, especially when a family has to deal with a poor prognosis and the possible loss of one parent.

Early menopause is now becoming a recognized long-term complication of chemotherapy given in adolescence (Marsden and Hacker 2003). Young adult cancer survivors are often advised to wait two years following the completion of treatment before trying to conceive, when health prospects become brighter. There is also evidence to suggest that teen-cancer-survivors exhibit delayed sexual maturity and first sexual experiences occur later than their peers (Kokkonen et al. 1997). These factors combine to limit duration of potential childbearing years. Communication concerning a shortening of reproductive years could serve to decrease psychological distress in the future by giving a survivor the correct facts to make an informed choice.

Even when a survivor has preserved fertility, they may feel extremely cautious about having children. One study suggested that 16 per cent of survivors had diminished childbearing desire, which they attributed to their cancer experience (Schover et al. 1999). This confirms early research by Koocher and O'Malley (1981) who demonstrated that teen-cancer-survivors with preserved fertility were less likely than their siblings and peers to produce children. This may be due to several factors including worry about congenital malformations or future health of offspring. However, another question that may cross the minds of survivors is that of pregnancy triggering a possible fatal relapse with the prospect of leaving a child motherless or fatherless. This is the question we shall consider next.

Question three: will pregnancy affect my cancer?

34 years old: one year after my second child's birth

> It's come back. I've relapsed – a secondary in my lung. I need major
> surgery and I am very sick. I might die. Bethany was one year old
> last month. And now my biggest fear? She may not even remember
> me. Nobody told me this could happen. My cancer was 17 years ago
> and I thought I was *cured*. But now it all makes sense and I can see
> what has happened. The doctor showed me a chest x-ray taken five
> years ago, when Adam was two years old. There it was – an
> embryonic secondary, just a tiny grain of salt but I could see it
> nonetheless. That's when my chest began to get bad – I just thought
> it was asthma. Then I had the two miscarriages and afterwards my
> breathing got so much worse. Then I became pregnant with
> Bethany and since then it's been one chest infection after another
> and now I know why. The secondary was there all the time growing
> alongside my babies, developing into a fully fledged killer and now
> the enemy has been unleashed and I have to fight it again, not just
> for me but for my children. I keep thinking how could I be so stupid
> not to see the link – but then even if I had, would I have chosen my
> own life or chosen to give them life? And I know that even if I die
> because of it, I have created life and so I shall live on in them. But I
> am desperate for her to remember me.

One reason cited by cancer survivors for choosing not to have children is the
fear that pregnancy will induce a relapse. Most relapses occur within the
first two years following diagnosis and therefore clinicians advise a two-
year disease-free interval before trying to conceive. There is evidence to
suggest that women misinterpret this, believing pregnancy causes relapse.
Huge publicity surrounding breast cancer and possible links to hormone
treatments may exaggerate these fears. Current evidence does not support
this and pregnancy is considered to be reasonably safe following most forms
of cancer (Agarwal *et al.* 1995; Palermo *et al.* 1995). Despite this, it would
seem that women are worrying unnecessarily and possibly refraining from
motherhood. For example, Schover's (1999) study showed that 17 per cent
of women worried that pregnancy could induce relapse. Only 33 per cent of
the sample had received advice about the health risks of pregnancy. This
leads us to conclude that correct information is not reaching survivors,
resulting in an overly pessimistic outlook. Survivors may well extrapolate
misleading information gleaned from the media to their own situations and

draw the wrong conclusions. Obtaining the correct information allows survivors to make an informed choice.

Conversely, after many years of being disease-free, a large number of survivors become lost to follow-up, meaning that our information about this cohort of childbearing survivors is incomplete. More high-quality longitudinal studies looking at the long-term psycho-social functioning of survivors would add to our understanding in this area. Follow-up could also be used to educate survivors in pre-conception health, inform women of the risks of miscarriage, premature birth and low birthweight babies, and provide reassurance concerning their children's future health as well as liaison with obstetricians dealing with higher risk pregnancies. Maintaining women in follow-up throughout childbearing years provides an enormous opportunity to carry out surveillance and obtain further data concerning the risks of pregnancy. Increased contact with oncology services at this stage of life may well provide answers to many anxiety-provoking questions.

Question four: what about my children?

Survivors worry greatly about their offspring's risk of inheriting cancer. Studies have shown that this is the greatest source of concern amongst survivors (American Society for Reproductive Medicine 1995; Stephen and Chandra 1998). This occurs even in situations where cancer type is not part of an inherited syndrome, despite reassuring evidence to the contrary (Green et al. 2003). At present, no increased risk of cancer in survivors' offspring has been demonstrated and yet amongst cancer survivors, a significantly higher rate of medically induced abortion has been shown to exist, which may reflect the degree of parental anxiety concerning a child developing cancer (Green et al. 2002, 2003). Other attitudinal surveys have shown that 42 per cent of survivors worry that their offspring have a higher risk of contracting cancer (Schover et al. 1999). The research conducted to date does not bear out these fears and, once again, it would seem that many young survivors are misinformed.

With genetically inherited cancer syndromes, the whole debate about pre-natal diagnosis presents difficult ethical questions. This topic is beyond the scope of this chapter and the reader is referred to Schover's excellent review of the topic (Schover 1999).

Current research shows that the vast majority of survivors view themselves positively as parents. Many survivors give account of a greater appreciation of life after cancer and, when fertility has been questioned in the past, subsequent children may be regarded as particularly precious. Surviving cancer and the accompanying treatment may also lead to increased resourcefulness, resilience and psychological growth. Although cancer survivors are less likely to become parents (Koocher and O'Malley 1981), it may be that they acquire better parenting skills.

36 years old: 18 months after my relapse

> Sports day dawns bright and sunny. I sit with my friends waiting for my kids' races. Last week my scans were clear – no cancer anywhere. Today I am celebrating with my friends so our ice-box contains strawberries and a bottle of wine. I overhear a bored dad saying, 'I hate sports day, don't you?' Immediately I think back to last year when my cancer was at its worst and I sat through sports day crying for the children I might not see grow up. But now things are different and I am 'all-clear'. Today, the sun seems hotter, the grass greener and the cries of happy children never more joyful. Today, sports day seems the most wonderful occasion ever and I laugh out loud when I see Adam jumping his way to third place. Winning Olympic gold could not beat this! Today I make a promise to myself: I shall never miss another sports day or any of my children's precious days. I shall aim for every sports day and remember my survival on this day. This year – this sports day – I am seeing my children grow a little older. 'Come on,' I say to my friends, 'third place – let's celebrate!'

Survivors usually reach the point where they need and want to tell their children something about their previous cancer experience. This may be precipitated by a relapse with need for further treatment, curiosity about hospital appointment attendance, residual physical disability, scars, or an awareness of heightened parental anxiety. I am not aware of any research that has looked at the attitudes or difficulties experienced by survivors reaching this stage of survivorship: the first large cohort of parenting survivors has only just 'come of age'. The amount of information a child needs and desires will depend upon their age, personality and development. A five-year-old child's understanding of illness and the anxiety surrounding it is very different from that of a 12-year-old. A younger child will see illness in terms of separation from a parent, whereas an older child will have developed a more abstract form of thinking with a deeper understanding that illness may result in death. This may produce a higher level of emotional distress. In the same way as a cancer survivor develops and matures in their understanding of cancer, so too do the offspring of survivors.

Cancer is like no other illness in that the word itself evokes fears of extreme suffering and premature death. Children may hear parents or friends talking about cancer in negative ways, resulting in wrong perceptions. Most children's experiences of cancer will be witnessed in grandparents or elderly neighbours who may well have had a debilitating illness or died. This can provoke extreme fear in children extrapolating the experience and applying it to a parent. The child may communicate this to the parent or may present with behavioural difficulties or regressive patterns such as bedwetting. It is important to use simple and honest explanation, using words, information and images in keeping with the child's age. Withholding information or giving incorrect information may lead to mistrust and subsequent emotional difficulty.

Bethany, five years old, four years after my relapse

> 'Mummy, Megan's grandpa died yesterday and she is very sad. She cried in class and Miss gave her a cuddle.' Bethany's face is pinched and worried and my heart lurches ominously.
>
> 'What did he die from darling?'
>
> 'Cancer. He was very old.' She pauses and I know she wants to ask more. 'Mummy, you had cancer didn't you?'
>
> 'Yes I did.'
>
> 'So...are you going to die soon?' Then she looks at me and her lip is trembling and her eyes are brimming with tears and my heart breaks for her. 'My friend said you will die like Megan's grandpa because you had cancer and then you will go away.' And now her tears fall and she sobs. 'I don't want you to go away and leave me!' I want to cry too because I know how much pain she feels for I have felt it before her. But I cannot cry because she needs me to be strong. I have done this before: told Adam at about the same age, on a sunny walk home from school. We got through and now he understands. I take a deep breath, pray for inspiration and explain to my little daughter about living with cancer. But somewhere inside me I feel it is so unfair because she is so young and should not have to face this, should not have to be frightened. So I hold her hand tightly and give her my strength and bring her with me on this journey of survival.

As a child grows and develops, their reaction to a parent's cancer will change. It is important to give the child opportunities to express this as they develop. As children age, they may want to be included more in discussions and occasions such as follow-up visits, particularly as they approach teenage years. The importance of check-up visits will be recognized, and reassurance of clear results needed. Children may begin to worry about contracting cancer because a parent has suffered: again explanation and reassurance will be required. Conversations that cancer 'runs in families', occurring in playgrounds and classrooms, need correction.

Children's defence mechanisms will vary as much as those of their parents. One child may deal with a parent's cancer by using denial, another by displacement of anxiety and another by rationalization. These defences will vary over time and with maturity. It may be that, during particularly stressful times, a child will revert to denial, seeming to know nothing about an illness that has been previously acknowledged. It may emerge that children of survivors seek to explain illness of a parent in the same way as a survivor and are drawn to caring professions and cancer causes.

Parenting as a survivor is not all about stressful situations. The concept of post-traumatic growth includes enhanced enjoyment of life and this can impact positively upon a survivor's children. The enhanced pleasure at seeing children grow up must surely be a two-way process with a consequent greater appreciation of family for the child. Living with the chronic illness of a parent may encourage offspring to become more caring, compassionate individuals with less prejudice against those not so fortunate. Resilience and resourcefulness in offspring may be enhanced. Children of survivors may develop deeper emotional and spiritual awareness as a result of the need to consider issues related to survival.

It will be necessary, over the years ahead, to ascertain the emotional and psychological health of our 'second generation survivors' in addition to their physical well-being if we are to obtain a complete picture of the impact of cancer on the transition to parenthood.

Adam, 11 years old, five years after my relapse

I get upset when I think about my mum having cancer because my mum can't run and stuff. When my mum has her anniversary or check-up I get worried thinking she might get ill again and when I was nine I cried in the playground but I didn't tell anyone because my friends wouldn't understand. But it is amazing my mum survived and all her doctors thought she wouldn't make it. Something told me she was going to be okay all the way through. I think my dad loves my mum more because of what she has been through and me and my sister respect my mum more because she acts likes a normal person with two legs, cycling and going to the gym. I'm more sensitive and loving and I think I am a stronger person because of what mum and me have been through emotionally. God has come closer to me because of my mum's illness.

Conclusion

I have attempted in this chapter to draw together relevant research and my own experiences to enhance our understanding of the problems facing the cancer survivor and the transition to parenthood. I believe this is an area ripe for research and one that can contribute to a better psychological outcome for survivors, significantly enhancing quality of life. Improved and effective communication throughout the cancer journey, a multi-disciplinary approach to long-term follow-up, as well as maintaining survivors in follow-up and referring them to experts for advice and reassurance, are areas that need to be addressed. There are many aspects of survivorship that are evolving as 'new experiences', presenting the need for ongoing research. Listening to survivors' narratives is one way in which we can discover both the positive growth and stressful challenges that inevitably accompany survivorship.

Note

1 My heartfelt thanks to my courageous and precious children, Adam and Bethany, for sharing their stories and experiences in this chapter, which is dedicated to them.

Part Four

Voices

Unintended Catharsis Through Intended Art

Dan Savage

As an artist, I was already using images of myself before I experienced illness at first hand. However, this took on a new dimension when, during my second year of a Fine Art degree, my diagnosis and treatment for testicular cancer necessitated a period of leave from university. During chemotherapy, I kept a sketchbook of pencil drawings in which I recorded much of the emotion and trauma of my treatment. When I had completed my treatment, I created a body of work based on my experience. I used two media, charcoal on paper and red enamel on transparent plastic, and both also incorporated print, text and handwriting.

During my illness, I may have become introspective. My sketchbook meticulously documented my illness. It contained self-portraits drawn at a time when I was feeling vulnerable and weak. Some sketches were done with my left hand because I was having chemotherapy in my right hand. When I look at these sketches, the trauma that I was experiencing at that time floods back. It is likely that my subconscious intention at the time was to find catharsis. I made use of the poignancy of some of the pictures in my later work. In order that I should preserve this rawness, I often used facsimiles of the drawings to allow the illness to communicate to the viewer but in a larger, retrospective context, transforming them from a raw material into art. In my final body of work, the pictures from my sketchbook added emotion but the emotions were no longer painful because they were being used in a different context, where my concerns were in the creation of art (see Figure 1).

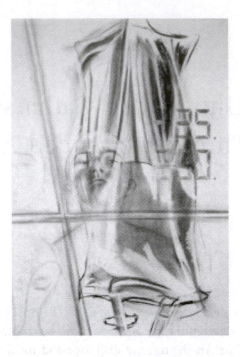

Figure 1 *Drip*, 2003, Dan Savage, charcoal on paper with printmaking

In a conversation with a fellow student, I acknowledged that making art-work about my illness seemed like an automatic thing to do. At the time, it seemed that if my work were to progress without any reference to cancer, I would have been denying the fact that I had been ill at all. Instead I accepted it and used it for inspiration. The final work did not just contain references to my illness but embraced it fully, but in a processed rather than a raw state.

At no point in the making of this work did I consciously seek catharsis, although when I look back at my work now, I see that its creation did have cathartic value. My need to keep drawing while receiving treatment was more for the sake of catharsis than for the sake of art. However, my seem-ingly rational intention at the time was to create art that continued on from the work I was producing prior to my illness. At that time I was interested in work that explored the role of the individual in a society saturated with tex-tual and image references. The individual's relationship with society was one of both anonymity and manipulation. The cancer work similarly por-trayed the plight of the individual – the anonymity experienced during ill-ness and the way in which life is governed by disease and treatment. The techniques used at this time combined printmaking and enamel paint on transparent plastic, enabling me to present several layers which acted as a metaphor for the layers of self. This medium was relevant for the work on cancer also since, during illness, an individual's life operates on different levels. At times, the individual may experience anonymity, while at other times they may be self-absorbed. The layers may also represent levels of consciousness and knowledge. The inclusion of relevant text in my work encourages the viewer to read it and piece together factual information from my experience.

The inclusion of text in artwork inevitably fixes the meaning of the work, making any loose interpretation of a piece unlikely and helping the illness to communicate more than the art (see Figure 2).

A fellow art student who knew my background both in terms of my previous work and my illness resisted accepting the work for its cathartic value or even as a documentation of my illness, remarking 'I don't see the illness in that work...I see you the artist' and later saying 'I am more interested in

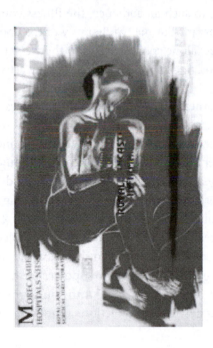

Figure 2 *Chop*, **2003, Dan Savage, enamel on PVC plastic film with printmaking**

what comes out of the illness, how it has changed your life.' This suggests that I was making the artwork for its own sake and that it could be appreciated in that way. A similar comment was made by a nurse at a presentation I gave about my art in which I had discussed the illness at length because of the medical audience. He questioned my approach as an artist, suggesting that, by being concerned with using my art to present my illness to this audience, I had not given sufficient weight to the visual values of the work. My art student colleague saw the work purely aesthetically, at the same time acknowledging that the illness helped in the creation of the art. It is worth comparing her response, as an art student, with those from outside the art world. Members of the medical profession and a lady who had experienced similar treatment for cancer brought with them a greater knowledge of the illness. Some found the work to be cathartic for them, and many recognized that it could have been cathartic for me. Yet for them, any desire to see the work as art was less significant than their interest in my response to the illness. It would seem that for these viewers, the catharsis that I experienced during the making of the art was almost more important than its value as art. This suggests that, to such an audience, the illness communicates more to the viewer than the art. For me, while my work is about cancer, I do not think that the illness alone communicates to the viewer, but I acknowledge that it has a function not only as the subject of my artwork, but also as the catalyst.

Unlike some other artists portraying their illness experience, I dealt with my illness in my work in a non-confrontational way. I was not angry with anyone or with the system, nor did I feel undermined in any way. I was not tense but rather accepting of the situation. Although I would concede that I am probably a self-obsessed artist. For that body of work at least, I approached my work as an artist, partly because I was an art student creating work for assessment. That said, I hope that my work exists on two levels, appealing to the health profession because of its subject matter and frank but ordered approach to cancer, and to the art world, for its artistic merit. People from both groups have said how powerful the end result was. My desire to create art was primary, and with hindsight I see that catharsis was definitely a catalyst in its production, although it was not a conscious starting block.

Orchid

Jen King

Explanation bringing release in form,
liberating without comfort
for the loss of things expected as norm.
Infinite consequences form microscopic fault,
on body, mind and life.

Although nurturing love has made me blessed,
cherishing and accepting,
Peace itself may have been my behest –
Self-ostracized, deprecatory, denying
in bitterness of soul.

Exotic plant, your beauty and aroma grows despite what cannot be:
no potential for other, pure femininity you know.
Do not wither, but resolve to blossom
Consider – **A**ccept – **I**nvert – **S**trengthen

Written by a woman living with Complete Androgen Insensitivity Syndrome (CAIS) and reproduced here under a pseudonym with her permission.

From One Parent to Another

Jane Davies

There are many, many different reasons for infertility and here is my family's experience. It will resonate with some of you and not with others. So hold that in your mind as I tell you my story.

We found out by chance that our son was almost certainly infertile when he was just 16. We were told by the experts not to tell him because, they said, 16 isn't a good time to tell a young man that he's probably infertile. Now I absolutely agree with them that it isn't a good time, but is 17 any better? As an 18th birthday present? When he's first engaged? Yes it's a bad time, but no other time was better as far as my husband and I were concerned. So we decided to tell him. It was partly because of that and partly because our family way of coping with things is to be up-front and honest with each other. When you want to tell somebody something, it does depend a little bit on how your family operates. If you tend to be secret and introverted then it's difficult to make an exception. But for us it was right to tell him, and he coped brilliantly. I coped far less well. I felt great pain, and enormous guilt – had I done something wrong? Was it my fault? I'd had a miscarriage and gone straight on and conceived him. Nobody told me that I ought to wait. It was a difficult pregnancy and I very nearly died when I had him because the placenta wasn't right. Whether that had any effect I don't know, but I carried that guilt and I do still. It's one of the things about being a parent: we think that we care for our children logically and lovingly, but of course we don't. As I became over-protective, my son found it hard. As he grew up, he coped far better than I did.

Now this might have happened anyway. Quite often a pretty strong Mum (as I think I was) can have quite a difficult time with an equally strong young man as he grows through later teens! I don't know whether the infertility affected it or not but it seemed to me that it did. I think I finally came to terms with it because of my daughter-in-law. She was the one who healed it for me. When we were talking after they were engaged and I said about children, I can always remember her looking at me and saying: 'But he's the one I love, he's the one I want to marry.' She loved him for himself not for the genes he could give to their children. I was then able to look at my son with different eyes. That makes a huge difference.

It's often somebody outside who helps us. I'm not underestimating what it is to be infertile, but I came to realize that it's not the most important thing in life. Whether your child has an illness or a disability or is infertile – whatever it is – you need to keep a sense of proportion. Though infertility is a very important thing, it's not the whole picture and we need to remember that.

My son and daughter-in-law have two lovely children now through using donor conception treatment and I have five grandchildren altogether. If somebody had said to me before about donor conception, I think I would have said that I had reservations. I had always got pregnant so easily and it seemed alien to think about using medical treatment. I worried that it might solve one set of issues but create another lot to face, such as issues around identity and how to tell the child. But with all things where your children are involved, you look at it afresh and remember that nothing in life is ever straightforward. That was what they wanted, I love them, so no more questions from my way of looking at it. Their children are my grandchildren as much as any of the others. Do I feel differently about them to the other grandchildren? No. Do I feel differently about them in any other way? Yes, but only because I feel differently about all my children and all my grandchildren. I have a unique relationship with each of them, but it's not to do with the manner of their conception.

We didn't actually tell anyone else about our son's infertility because we felt it was his story, not ours. I found that extraordinarily difficult. I longed to be able to discuss it with others, including close family, because that's the way I am. Once he gave me permission then I was able to, but it was one of the hardest things to respect. But my husband and I felt certain that, at 16, it was his story and not for us to tell.

There is a temptation sometimes when a child is very ill, or with a child who seems so precious because of all you've gone through, to make that child special because of that. But all children are special because of what they are, not where they came from or what they're going through. It's that specialness and the uniqueness of the relationship that you build up that every child deserves.

For me, coping with my son's infertility hasn't always been easy and it's still painful. While it's important to spend time thinking about what's happening now and in the past from time to time, it's also important to use those experiences as parents and grandparents to learn and move on. Having children gives us a chance to face again our attitudes, to rethink them. We think that we shape children's lives, but of course they shape ours just as much. Parenting is a two-way process.

Happy in Her Own Skin

Sarah Clough

Mum and Dad told me I had Turner Syndrome when I was 15. They had just found out themselves. My first reaction and gut instinct was 'What man will want me now?' Mum and Dad reassured me that any man worth his 'salt' would want me for me not for what I may or may not be able to give him.

So the process of coming to terms with infertility had begun. OK, so I was infertile but did it change me? I had Turner Syndrome but was I really that different? Yes, deep down I was, my chromosomes were different. But what did that mean? Aren't we all individuals? Don't we all have our own 'foibles' that make us different from one another? I gradually came to accept I may not like Turner's or being infertile but it was one of those things that made me...me. It was part of me, part of my personality.

Life continued; after all at 15, children didn't seem that important. I was not ready to think about whether I might have wanted children. But that choice had been taken away.

I completed my GCSEs, 'A' Levels, and went off to university. Did the normal things a teenager might do. Started a career. I was more determined that I would make a success of my life; this 'thing' wouldn't be responsible for destroying my hopes, dreams and ambitions.

Relationships started to come and go. Did they need to know? When did they need to know? Through friends I met Martin; after a while I realized this would be a 'serious' relationship. I decided I needed to tell him about the Turner's and not being able to have children. Would he reject me? Could he accept it? Would that be the end of the relationship? He told me it was me he was interested in and if that meant being childless or looking at other options such as adoption then so be it.

Four years later we married. I married him knowing he was fully accepting me for me and that was all of me 'warts (or Turner's) and all'.

Six years after meeting the man my Mum and Dad described, I gave birth to our son. No miracles, just a long slog at IVF and egg donation.

So what do people see when they look at 'me' now from the outside in? Hopefully, it's a young mum happy in her own skin.

References

Ackard, D.M. and Neumark-Sztainer, D. (2001) 'Health care information sources for adolescents: Age and gender differences on use, concerns, and needs.' *Journal of Adolescent Health 29*, 3, 170–176.

Agarwal, A., Shekarriz, M., Sidhu, R.K. and Thomas, A.J. (1995) 'Optimum abstinence time for cryopreservation of semen in cancer patients.' *Journal of Urology 86*, 4, 697–709.

Ahmad, N.H. (2003) 'Assisted reproduction – Islamic views on the science of procreation.' *Eubios Journal of Asian and International Bioethics 13*, 59–60.

Ahmad, W.I.U. (1996) 'Family obligations and social change in Asian families.' In W.I.U. Ahmad and K. Atkin (eds) *'Race' and Community Care*. Buckingham: Open University Press.

Ahmad, W.I.U. (2000) 'Introduction.' In W.I.U. Ahmad (ed.) *Ethnicity, Disability and Chronic Illness*. Buckingham: Open University Press.

Ahmad, W.I.U., Atkin, K. and Chamba, R. (2000) 'Causing havoc among their children: Parental and professional perspectives on consanguinity and childhood disability.' In W.I.U. Ahmad (ed.) *Ethnicity, Disability and Chronic Illness*. Buckingham: Open University Press.

Ahmad, W.I.U., Atkin, K. and Jones, L. (2002) 'Young Asian deaf people and their families: negotiating relationships and identities.' *Social Science and Medicine 55*, 10, 1757–1769.

Alan Guttmacher Institute (AGI) (2001) *Teenage Sexual and Reproductive Behavior in Developed Countries: Can More Progress Be Made?* New York: AGI.

Alderson, A. (2004) 'Girls as young as 14 demand NHS fertility treatment.' *The Telegraph* 4 July.

Alderson, P. (1994) *Children's Consent to Surgery*. Buckingham: Open University Press.

Alderson, P. (2000) *Young Children's Rights*. London: Jessica Kingsley Publishers.

Ali, N., Neal, R. and Atkin, K. (2003) *Communication between GPs and South Asian Patients: Final Report to Northern and Yorkshire Regional Health Authority*. Leeds: Centre for Research in Primary Care.

Allenye, J. and Thomas, V.J. (1994) 'The management of sickle cell crisis pain as experienced by patients and their carers.' *Journal of Advanced Nursing 19*, 4, 725–732.

Almodin, C.G., Minguetti-Camara, V.C., Meister, H., Ferreira, J.O., Franco, R.L., Cavalcante, A.A., Radaelli, M.R., Bahls, A.S., Moron, A.F. and Murta, C.G. (2004) 'Recovery of fertility after grafting of cryopreserved germinative tissue in female rabbits following radiotherapy.' *Human Reproduction 19*, 1287–1293.

American Academy of Pediatrics, Committee on Pediatric AIDS (1999) 'Disclosure of illness status to children and adolescents with HIV infection.' *Pediatrics 103*, 1, 164–166.

American Society for Reproductive Medicine (1995) *Fertility After Cancer Treatment: A Guide for Patients*. Birmingham, AL: American Society for Reproductive Medicine.

Anionwu, E. and Atkin, K. (2001) *The Politics of Sickle Cell and Thalassaemia*. Buckingham: Open University Press.

Aslam, I., Fishel, S., Moore, H., Dowell, K. and Thornton, S. (2000) 'Fertility preservation of boys undergoing anti-cancer therapy: A review of the existing situation and prospects for the future.' *Human Reproduction 15*, 10, 2154–2159.

Association of London Government (2000) *Sick of Being Excluded: Improving the Health and Care of London's Black and Minority Ethnic Communities*. London: Association of London Government.

Ataya, K., Rao, L.V., Lawrence, E. and Kimmel, R. (1995) 'Luteinizing hormone-releasing hormone agonist inhibits cyclophosphamide-induced ovarian follicular depletion in rhesus monkeys.' *Biology of Reproduction 52*, 365–372.

Atkin, K. (2004) 'Primary health care and South Asian populations: Institutional racism, policy and practice.' In S. Ali and K. Atkin (eds) *South Asian Populations and Primary Health Care: Meeting the Challenges.* Oxford: Radcliffe.

Atkinson, H.G., Apperley, J.F., Dawson, K., Goldman, J.M. and Winston, R.M. (1994) 'Successful pregnancy after allogeneic bone marrow transplantation for chronic myeloid leukaemia.' *Lancet 344*, 199.

Azar, S.T. and Rohrbeck, C.A. (1986) 'Child abuse and unrealistic expectations.' *Journal of Consulting and Clinical Psychology 54*, 867–868.

Bahadur, G., Chatterjee, R. and Ralph, D. (2000) 'Testicular tissue cryopreservation in boys: Ethical and legal issues.' *Human Reproduction 15*, 6, 1416–1420.

Bahadur, G., Ling, K.L.E., Hart, R., Ralph, D., Wafa, R., Ashraf, A.A., Jaman, N., Mahmud, S. and Oyede, A.W. (2002) 'Semen quality and cryopreservation in adolescent cancer patients.' *Human Reproduction 17*, 3157–3161.

Bahadur, G., Nahadur, G., Ozturk, O., Muneer, A., Wafa, R., Ashraf, A., Jaman, N., Patel, S., Oyede, A.W. and Ralph, D.J. (2005) 'Semen quality before and after gonadotoxic treatment.' *Human Reproduction 20*, 774–781.

Bahadur, G., Whelan, J., Ralph, D. and Hindmarsh, P. (2001) 'Gaining consent to freeze spermatozoa from adolescents with cancer: Legal, ethical and practical aspects.' *Human Reproduction 16*, 1, 188–193.

Bainton, V., Neylon, L., McGregor, L. and Stewart, P.M. (1999) *Long-term Effects of Congenital Adrenal Hyperplasia (Abstract).* Bristol: Society for Endocrinology.

Balen, A.H. (2001) 'Polycystic ovary syndrome and cancer.' *Human Reproduction Update 7*, 522–525.

Balen, A.H. (2004) 'Ovulation induction.' *Current Obstetrics & Gynaecology 14*, 261–268.

Balen, A.H., Conway, G.S., Kaltsas, G., Techatrasak, K., Manning, P.J., West, C. and Jacobs, H.S. (1995) 'Polycystic ovary syndrome: The spectrum of the disorder in 1741 patients.' *Human Reproduction 10*, 2107–2111.

Balen, A.H., Creighton, S.M., Davies, M.C., MacDougall, J. and Stanhope, R. (eds) (2004) *Paediatric and Adolescent Gynaecology: Management of Developmental Abnormalities and Disorders.* Cambridge: Cambridge University Press.

Balen, R. (2000) 'Listening to children with cancer.' *Children & Society 14*, 3, 159–167.

Balen, R., Blyth, E., Calabretto, H., Fraser, C., Horrocks, C. and Manby, M. (2006) 'Involving children in health and social research – "human becomings" or "active beings"?' *Childhood 13*, 1, 29–48.

BAPS (2001) *Statement of the British Association of Paediatric Surgeons Working Party on the Surgical Management of Children Born with Ambiguous Genitalia July 2001.* www.baps.org.uk, accessed on 25 July 2005.

Barry, M. (2001) *Challenging Transitions: Young People's Views and Experiences of Growing Up.* London: Save the Children.

Baskin, L.S., Ero, I.A., Li, Y.W., Liu, W.H., Kurzrock, E. and Cunha, G.R. (1999) 'Anatomical studies of the human clitoris.' *The Journal of Urology 162*, 1015–1120.

Bateman, A., Brown, D. and Pedder, J. (eds) (2000) *Introduction to Psychotherapy: An Outline of Psychodynamic Principles and Practice.* Third Edition. London: Routledge.

Bath, L.E., Anderson, R.A., Critchley, H.O.D., Kelnar, C.J.H. and Wallace, W.H.B. (2001) 'Hypothalamic-pituitary-ovarian dysfunction after prepubertal chemotherapy and cranial irradiation for acute leukaemia.' *Human Reproduction 16*, 1838–1844.

Bath, L.E., Wallace, W.H.D., Shaw, M.P., Fitzpatrick, C. and Anderson, R.A. (2003) 'Depletion of ovarian reserve in young women after treatment for cancer in childhood: Detection by anti-Müllerian hormone, inhibin B and ovarian ultrasound.' *Human Reproduction 18*, 11, 2368–2374.

Bekker, H.L., Hewison, J. and Thornton, J.G. (2003) 'Understanding why decision aids work: Linking process with outcome.' *Patient Education and Counseling 50*, 323–329.

Bekker, H., Thornton, J.G., Airey, C.M., Connelly, J.B., Hewison, J. and Robinson, M.B. (1999) 'Informed decision making: An annotated bibliography and systematic review.' *Health Technology Assessment 3*, 1, 278–279.

Berenbaum, S.A. and Bailey, J.M. (2003) 'Effects on gender identity of prenatal androgens and genital appearance: Evidence from girls with Congenital Adrenal Hyperplasia.' *The Journal of Clinical Endocrinology & Metabolism 88*, 3, 1102–1106.

Berg, B.J., Wilson, J.F. and Weingartner, P.J. (1991) 'Psychological sequelae of infertility treatment: The role of gender and sex-role identification.' *Social Science and Medicine 33*, 1071–1080.

Betensky, M. (1987) 'Phenomenology of therapeutic art expression and art therapy.' In J. Rubin (ed.) *Approaches to Art Therapy: Theory and Technique.* New York: Brunner Mazel.

Bhakta, P., Katbamna, S. and Parker, G. (2000) 'South Asian carers' experiences of primary health care teams.' In W.I.U. Ahmad (ed.) *Ethnicity, Disability and Chronic Illness.* Buckingham: Open University Press.

Bharadwaj, A. (2003) 'Why adoption is not an option in India: The visibility of infertility, the secrecy of donor insemination, and other cultural complexities.' *Social Science and Medicine 56*, 1867–1880.

Bick, D., Sherins, R.J., Heye, B., Pike, L., Crawford, J., Maddalena, A., Incerti, B., Pragliola, A. and Meitinger, T. (1992) 'Brief report: Intragenic deletion of the Kalig-1 gene in Kallmann's syndrome.' *New England Journal of Medicine 326*, 1752–1755.

Blackhall, F.H., Atkinson, A.D., Maaya, M.B., Ryder, W.D., Horne, G., Brison, D.R., Lieberman, B.A. and Radford, J.A. (2002) 'Semen cryopreservation, utilisation and reproductive outcome in men treated for Hodgkin's disease.' *British Journal of Cancer 12*, 381–384.

Blacklay, A., Eiser, C. and Ellis, A. (1998) 'Development and evaluation of an information booklet for adult survivors of cancer in childhood.' *Archives of Disease in Childhood 78*, 4, 340–344 (April).

Blackless, M., Charuvastra, A., Derryck, A., Fausto-Sterling, A., Lauzanne, K. and Lee, E. (2000) 'How sexually diamorphic are we? Review and synthesis.' *American Journal of Human Biology 12*, 151–166.

Blank, J. (ed.) (1993) *Femalia.* San Francisco: Down There Press.

Blatt, J. (1999) 'Pregnancy outcome in long-term survivors of childhood cancer.' *Medical and Pediatric Oncology 33*, 29–33.

Blumenfeld, Z., Avivi, I., Linn, S., Epelbaum, R., Ben-Shahar, M. and Haim, N. (1996) 'Prevention of irreversible chemotherapy-induced ovarian damage in young women with lymphoma by a gonadotrophin-releasing hormone agonist in parallel to chemotherapy.' *Human Reproduction 11*, 1620–1626.

Blyth, E. (1995) *Infertility and Assisted Conception: Practice Issues for Counsellors.* Birmingham: British Association of Social Workers.

Blyth, E. and Moore, R. (2001) 'Involuntary childlessness and stigma.' In T. Mason (ed.) *Stigma and Social Exclusion in Healthcare.* London: Routledge.

Boekelheide, K., Schoenfeld, H.A., Hall, S.J., Weng, C.C., Shetty, G., Leith, J., Harper, J., Sigman, M., Hess, D.L. and Meistrich, M.L. (2005) 'Gonadotropin-releasing hormone antagonist (Cetrorelix) therapy fails to protect nonhuman primates (*macaca arctoides*) from radiation-induced spermatogenic failure.' *Journal of Andrology 26 ,222–234.*

Borini, A., Bonu, M.A., Coticchio, G., Bianchi, V., Cattoli, M. and Flamigni, C. (2004) 'Pregnancies and births after oocyte cryopreservation.' *Fertility and Sterility 18,* 601–605.

Borland, M., Laybourn, A., Hill, M. and Brown, J. (1998) *Middle Childhood: The Perspectives of Children and Parents.* London: Jessica Kingsley Publishers.

Borzekowski, D.L.G. and Rickert, V.I. (2001) 'Adolescents, the internet, and health: Issues of access and content.' *Journal of Applied Developmental Psychology 22,* 1, 49–59.

Bowler, I. (1993) 'They are not the same as us: Midwives' stereotypes of South Asian maternity patients.' *Sociology of Health and Illness 15,* 2, 157–178.

Bradby, H. (2003) 'Describing ethnicity in health research.' *Ethnicity and Health 8,* 1, 5–13.

Bradshaw, J. (ed.) (2002) *The Well-being of Children in the UK.* London: Save the Children.

Bradshaw, J., Finch, N. and Miles, J.N.V. (2005) 'Deprivation and variation in teenage conceptions and abortions in England.' *Journal of Family Planning and Reproductive Health Care 31,* 1, 15–19.

Brannen, J., Dodd, K., Oakley, A. and Storey, P. (1994) *Young People, Health and Family Life.* Buckingham: Open University Press.

Brinster, R.L. and Zimmermann, J.W. (1994) 'Spermatogenesis following male germ cell transplantation.' *Proceedings of the National Academy of Sciences USA 91,* 11298–11302.

Bristol Royal Infirmary Inquiry (2001) *Learning from Bristol: The Report of the Inquiry into Children's Heart Surgery at the Bristol Royal Infirmary 1984–1995.* Norwich: The Stationery Office.

Brooks-Gunn, J. and Furstenberg, F.F. (1989) 'Adolescent sexual behavior.' *American Psychologist 44,* 2, 249–257.

Broome, M.E. and Allegretti, C. (2001) 'Adolescent cancer patients: Sperm storage, consent and emotion.' *Human Reproduction 16,* 11, 2473.

Bunting, M. (2004) 'Family fortunes.' *Guardian Unlimited, The Guardian* 25 September.

Burr, J.A. and Bean, F.D. (1996) 'Racial fertility differences: The role of female employment and education in wanted and unwanted child bearing.' *Social Biology 43,* 3–4, 218–241.

Butt, J. and Mirza, K. (1996) *Social Care and Black Communities.* London: HMSO.

Byrne, J. (1999a) 'Infertility and premature menopause in childhood cancer survivors.' *Medical and Pediatric Oncology 33,* 24–28.

Byrne, J. (1999b) 'Long-term genetic and reproductive effects of ionizing radiation and chemotherapeutic agents on cancer patients and their offspring.' *Teratology 59,* 210–215.

Byrne, J., Fears, T.R., Mills, J.L., Zeltzer, L.K., Sklar, C., Meadows, A.T., Reaman, G.H. and Robison, L.L. (2004) 'Fertility of long-term male survivors of acute lymphoblastic leukemia diagnosed during childhood.' *Pediatric Blood and Cancer 42,* 364–372.

Byrne, J., Rasmussen, S.A., Steinhorn, S.C., Connelly, R.R., Myers, M.H., Lynch, C.F., Flannery, J., Austin, D.F., Holmes, F.F., Holmes, G.E., Strong, L.C. and Mulvihill, J.J. (1998) 'Genetic disease in offspring of long-term survivors of childhood and adolescent cancer.' *American Journal of Human Genetics 62,* 45–52.

Callan, V.J. (1982) 'How do Australians value children? A review and research update using the perceptions of parents and voluntarily childless adults.' *Australian and New Zealand Journal of Sociology 18,* 384–398.

Callan, V.J. (1983) 'Perceptions of parenthood and childlessness: A comparison of mothers and voluntarily childless wives.' *Population and Environment 6*, 179–189.

Callan, V.J. (1987) 'The personal and marital adjustment of mothers, voluntary and involuntary childless wives.' *Journal of Marriage and the Family 48*, 849–856.

Carmichael, C. and Alderson, J. (2004) 'Psychological care in disorders of sexual differentiation and determination.' In A.H. Balen, S.M. Creighton, M.C. Davies, J. MacDougall and R. Stanhope (eds) *Paediatric and Adolescent Gynaecology: Management of Developmental Abnormalities and Disorders.* Cambridge: Cambridge University Press.

Cartwright-Alcarese, F. (1995) 'Addressing sexual dysfunction following radiation therapy for a gynaecologic malignancy.' *Oncology Nursing Forum 22*, 1227–1232.

Carvel, J. (2000) 'More women delay starting their families.' *The Guardian* 21 June.

Cella, D. and Najavits, L. (1986) 'Denial of infertility in patients with Hodgkin's Disease.' *Psychosomatics 27*, 71.

Central Office of Research Ethics Committees (COREC) (2003) *Ethical Issues in Research in Children.* London: COREC.

Chamba, R., Ahmad, W.I.U., Hirst, M., Lawton, B. and Beresford, B. (1999) *On the Edge: A National Survey of Minority Ethnic Parents Caring for a Severely Disabled Child.* Bristol: Policy Press.

Chambas, K. (1991) 'Sexual concerns of adolescents with cancer.' *Journal of Pediatric Oncology Nursing 8*, 4, 165–172.

Chambers, D., van Loon, J. and Tincknell, E. (2004) 'Teachers' views of teenage sexual morality.' *British Journal of Sociology of Education 25*, 2, 563–571.

Chan, P.T., Palermo, G.D., Veeck, L.L., Rosenwaks, Z. and Schlegel, P.N. (2001) 'Testicular sperm extraction combined with intra-cytoplasmic sperm injection in the treatment of men with persistent azoospermia post-chemotherapy.' *Cancer 92*, 1632–1637.

Chattoo, S. and Ahmad, W.I.U. (2004) 'The meaning of cancer: Illness, biography and social identity.' In D. Kelleher and G. Leavey (eds) *Identity and Health.* London: Routledge.

Chattoo, S., Atkin, K. and McNeish, D. (2004) *Young People of Pakistani Origin and their Families: Implications for Providing Support to Young People and Their Families.* Ilford: Barnardos.

Chavez, L.R. (2004) 'A glass half empty: Latina reproduction and public discourse.' *Human Organisation*, Summer, 63, 2.

Chemes, H.E. (2001) 'Infancy is not a quiescent period of testicular development.' *Journal of Andrology 24*, 2–7.

Chesler, M. and Barbarin, O. (1984) 'Difficulties of providing help in a crisis: Relationships between parents of children with cancer and their friends.' *Journal of Social Issues 40*, 4, 113–134.

Chesler, M. and Barbarin, O. (1987) *Childhood Cancer and the Family.* New York: Brunner/Mazel.

Chesler, M., Weigers, M. and Lawther, T. (1992) 'How am I different? Perspectives for childhood cancer survivors on change and growth.' In D.M. Green and G. D'Angio (eds) *Late Effects of Treatment for Childhood Cancer.* New York: Wiley and Sons.

Clautour, S.E. and Moore, T.W. (1969) 'Attitudes of 12 year old children to present and future life roles.' *Human Development 12*, 4, 221–238.

CMEC (2001) *Determinants of Sexual Health.* Council of Ministers of Education Canada, available as a pdf file at www.cmec.ca, accessed 20 May 2005.

Cohen, L.F., di Sant'Agnese, P.A. and Freidlander, J. (1980) 'Cystic fibrosis and pregnancy: A national survey.' *Lancet 2*, 842–844.

Coleman, J. and Roker, D. (eds) (1998) *Teenage Sexuality: Health, Risk and Education*. London: Harwood.

Coley, R.L. and Chase-Lansdale, P.L. (1998) 'Adolescent pregnancy and parenthood: Recent evidences and future directions.' *American Psychologist 53*, 2, 152–166.

Commission for Racial Equality (2003) *Stakeholder Strategy Consultation: Health and Social Care*. London: CRE.

Condon, J.T., Donovan, J. and Corkindale, C.J. (2000) 'Australian adolescents' attitudes and beliefs concerning pregnancy, childbirth and parenthood: The development, psychometric testing and results of a new scale.' *Journal of Adolescence 24*, 729–742.

Connolly, J., Craig, W., Goldberg, A. and Pepler, D. (1999) 'Conceptions of cross-sex friendships and romantic relationships in early adolescence.' *Journal of Youth and Adolescence 28*, 4, 481–494.

Conway, G.S. (2001) 'Premature ovarian failure.' *British Medical Bulletin 56*, 643–649.

Cook, P. (1999) '"Will it hurt?" Children and medical settings.' In P. Milner and B. Carolin (eds) *Time to Listen to Children: Personal and Professional Communication*. London: Routledge.

Corker, M. and French, S. (1998) *Disability Discourse*. Buckingham: Open University Press.

Cottrell, D. (1996) *Social Networks and Social Influences in Adolescence*. London: Routledge.

Crawshaw, M., Glaser, A., Hale, J., Phelan, L. and Sloper, P. (2003) *A Study of the Decision Making Process Surrounding Sperm Storage for Adolescent Minors within Paediatric Oncology*. NHS Northern and Yorkshire Region: Research Report, available from M. Crawshaw, Dept. of Social Policy and Social Work, University of York.

Crawshaw, M.A., Glaser, A.W., Hale, J.K. and Sloper, P. (2004) 'Professionals' views on the issues and challenges arising from providing a fertility preservation service through sperm banking to teenage males with cancer.' *Human Fertility 7*, 1, 23–30.

Creighton, S.M. (2004) *Prevalence and Incidence of Child Abuse: International Comparisons*. London: National Society for the Prevention of Cruelty to Children, Research Report. Available from http://www.nspcc.org.uk/inform/Info_Briefing/PrevalenceAndIncidenceOfChildAbuse.asp.

Creighton, S.M. (2001) 'Surgery for intersex.' *Journal for the Royal Society of Medicine 94*, 218–220.

Creighton, S.M. and Minto, C.L. (2001) 'Managing intersex.' *British Medical Journal 323*, 1264–1265.

Creighton, S.M., Alderson, J., Brown, S. and Minto, C.L. (2002) 'Medical photography: Ethics, consent and the intersex patient.' *British Journal of Urology International 89*, 67–72.

Creighton, S.M., Minto, C.L. and Steele, S.J. (2001) 'Objective cosmetic and anatomical outcomes at adolescence of feminising surgery for ambiguous genitalia done in childhood.' *Lancet 358*, 124–125.

Critchley, H.O., Wallace, W.H., Shalet, S.M., Mamtora, H., Higginson, J. and Anderson, D.C. (1992) 'Abdominal irradiation in childhood: The potential for pregnancy.' *British Journal of Obstetrics and Gynaecology 99*, 392–394.

Crouch, N.S., Minto, C.L., Laio, L.M., Woodhouse, C.R. and Creighton, S.M. (2004) 'Genital sensation after feminizing genitoplasty for Congenital Adrenal Hyperplasia: A pilot study.' *British Journal of Urology International 93*, 135–138.

Cull, M. (2002) 'Treatment of intersex needs open discussion.' *British Medical Journal 324*, 919.

Cull, M.L. (2005) 'A support group's perspective.' *British Medical Journal, 330*, 7487, 341.

Culley, L., Rapport, F., Katbamna, S., Johnson, M. and Hudson, N. (2004) *A Study of the Provision of Infertility Services to South Asian Communities. Final Report prepared for NHS Executive Policy and Practice Research and Development Programme*. Leicester: De Montfort University.

Damani, M.N., Master, V., Meng, M.V., Burgess, C., Turek, P., Oates, R.D. and Masters, V. (2002) 'Post-chemotherapy ejaculatory azoospermia fatherhood with sperm from testis tissue with intracytoplasmic sperm injections.' *Journal of Clinical Oncology 20*, 888–890.

Davis, C.J., Davidson, R.M., Rodeck, C.H., Conway, G.S. (2000) 'X chromosome defects as a cause of idiopathic familial premature ovarian failure.' *British Journal of Obstetrics and Gynaecology 107*, 819.

de Bruin, J.P., Dorland, M., Spek, E.R., Posthuma, G., van Haaften, M., Looman, C.W. and te Velde, E.R. (2002) 'Ultrastructure of the resting ovarian follicle pool in healthy young women.' *Biology of Reproduction 66*, 1151–1160.

de Bruin, J.P., Dorland, M., Spek, E.R., Posthuma, G., van Haaften, M., Looman, C.W. and te Velde, E.R. (2004) 'Age-related changes in the ultrastructure of the resting follicle pool in human ovaries.' *Biology of Reproduction 70*, 419–424.

De Mas, P., Daudin, M., Vincent, M.C., Bourrouilou, G., Calvas, P., Mieusset, R. and Bujan, L. (2001) 'Increased aneuploidy in spermatozoa from testicular tumour patients after chemotherapy with cisplatin, etoposide and bleomycin.' *Human Reproduction 16*, 1204–1208.

Department of Health (DoH) (2000) *The Children Act Report 1995–1999*. London: HMSO.

Department of Health (DoH) (2001) *A Code of Practice for Tissue Banks: Providing Tissues of Human Origin for Therapeutic Purposes*. London: HMSO.

Department of Health (DoH) (2004a) *Best Practice Guidance for Doctors and Other Health Professionals on the Provision of Advice and Treatment to Young People Under 16 on Contraception, Sexual and Reproductive Health*. Available at www.dh.gov.uk, accessed 19 May 2005.

Department of Health (DoH) (2004b) *Consent – What You Have a Right to Expect. A Guide for Children and Young People*. London: HMSO.

Department of Health (DoH) (2004c) Press Release: 'Reid: Reducing NHS bureaucracy to release resources to the frontline.' 22 July, ref no: 2004/0271.

Diamond, M. (2000) 'Atypical gender identity development therapeutic models, philosophical and ethical issues.' Paper presented at Tavistock & Portman NHS Trust conference, 17–18 November, London.

Diamond, M. and Sigmundson, H.K. (1997) 'Management of intersexuality: Guidelines for dealing with individuals with ambiguous genitalia.' *Archives of Pediatrics & Adolescent Medicine 151*, 1046–1050.

DiCenso, A., Guyatt, G., Willan, A., Griffith, L. and Buske, L. (2002) 'Interventions to reduce unintended teenage pregnancies among adolescents: A systematic review of randomised controlled trials.' *British Medical Journal 324*, 7351, 1426.

DiClemente, R.J., Wingood, G.M., Sionean, C., Crosby, R., Harrington, K., Davies, S., Hook, E.W. 3rd and Oh, M.K. (2002) 'Association of adolescents' history of sexually transmitted disease (STD) and their current high-risk behavior and STD status: A case for intensifying clinic-based prevention efforts.' *Sexually Transmitted Diseases 29*, 9, 503–509.

Die-Trill, M. and Stuber, M.L. (1998) 'Psychological problems of curative cancer treatment.' In J.C. Holland (ed.) *Psycho-oncology*. New York: Oxford University Press.

Dixon-Woods, M., Young, B. and Heney, D. (1999) 'Partnerships with children.' *British Medical Journal 319*, 778–780.

Dodge, J.A., Morison, S., Lewis, P.A., Coles, C.S., Geddes, D., Russell, G., Littlewood, J.M. and Scott, M.T. (the UK CF survey management committee) (1997) 'Incidence, population and survival of cystic fibrosis in the United Kingdom.' *Archives of Disease in Childhood 77*, 493–496.

Dolgin, M.J., Somer, E., Buchvald, E. and Zaisov, R. (1999) 'Quality of life in adult survivors of childhood cancer.' *Social Work in Health Care 28*, 4, 31–43.

Donnelly, E.T., Steele, E.K., McClure, N. and Lewis, S. (2001) 'Assessment of DNA integrity and morphology of ejaculated spermatozoa from fertile and infertile men before and after cryopreservation.' *Human Reproduction 16*, 1191–1199.

Donnez, J., Dolmans, M.M., Demylle, D., Jadoul, P., Pirard, C., Squifflet, J., Martinez-Madrid, B. and van Langendonckt, A. (2004) 'Livebirth after orthotopic transplantation of cryopreserved ovarian tissue.' *Lancet 364*, 1405–1410.

Dudding, T., Wilcken, B., Burgess, B., Hambly, J. and Turner, G. (2000) 'Reproductive decisions after neonatal screening identifies cystic fibrosis.' *Archives of Disease in Childhood Fetal & Neonatal Edition 82*, F124–F127.

Dunkel-Schetter, C. and Lobel, M. (1991) 'Psychological reactions to infertility.' In L. Stanton and C. Dunkel-Schetter (eds) *Infertility: Perspectives from Stress and Coping Research.* New York: Plenum Press.

Edelmann, R.J., Humphrey, M. and Owens, D.J. (1994) 'The meaning of parenthood and couples' reactions to male infertility.' *British Journal of Medical Psychology 67*, 291–299.

Edenborough, F.P. (2002) 'Pregnancy in women with cystic fibrosis.' *Acta Obstetriciaet Gynecologica Scandinavica 81*, 689–692.

Edenborough, F.P., Mackenzie, W.E. and Stableforth, D.E. (2000) 'The outcome of 73 pregnancies in 55 women with cystic fibrosis in the UK 1977–1996.' *British Journal of Obstetrics and Gynaecology 107*, 254–261.

Editorial (1992) 'Congenital bilateral absence of the vas deferens and cystic fibrosis.' *Lancet 339*, 1328–1329.

Eiser, C. (1993) *Growing up with a Chronic Disease: The Impact on Children and their Families.* London: Jessica Kingsley Publishers.

Eiser, C. (1996) 'Children's knowledge of chronic disease and implications for education: A review.' In L.R. Schmidt, P. Schwenmezger, J.A. Weinman and S. Maes (eds) *Theoretical and Applied Aspects of Health Psychology.* New York: Harwood Academic Publishers.

Eiser, C. (1998) 'Practitioner review: Long-term consequences of childhood cancer.' *Journal of Child Psychology and Psychiatry 39*, 621–633.

Elad, P., Yagill, Y., Cohen, L.H. and Meller, I. (2003) 'A jeep trip with young adult cancer survivors: Lessons to be learned.' *Supportive Care in Cancer 11*, 4, 201–206.

Elsheikh, M., Dunger, D., Conway, G. and Wass, J. (2002) 'Turner's syndrome in adulthood.' *Endocrine Reviews 23*, 1, 120–140.

Erikson, E.H. (1950) *Childhood and Society.* New York: Norton.

Fabbri, R., Porcu, E., Marsella, T., Rocchetta, G., Venturoli, S. and Flamigni, C. (2001) 'Human oocyte cryopreservation: New perspectives regarding oocyte survival.' *Human Reproduction 16*, 411–416.

Faddy, M.J., Gosden, R.G., Gougeon, A., Richardson, S.J. and Nelson, J.F. (1992) 'Accelerated disappearance of ovarian follicles in mid-life: Implications for forecasting menopause.' *Human Reproduction 7*, 1342–1346.

Fair, A., Griffiths, K. and Osman, L.M. (2000) 'Attitudes to fertility among adults with cystic fibrosis in Scotland.' *Thorax 55*, 672–677.

Fauser, B., Tarlatzis, B., Chang, J., Azziz, R., Legro, R., Dewailly, D., Franks, S., Balen, A.H., Bouchard, P., Dahlgren, E., Devoto, L., Diamanti, E., Dunaif, A., Filicori, M., Homburg, R., Ibanez, L., Laven, J., Magoffin, D., Nestle, R.J., Norman, R., Pasquali, R., Pugeat, M., Strauss, J., Tan, S.L., Taylor, A., Wild, R. and Wild, S. (2004) 'The Rotterdam

ESHRE/ASRM-sponsored PCOS consensus workshop group. Revised 2003 consensus on diagnostic criteria and long-term health risks related to polycystic ovary syndrome (PCOS).' *Fertility and Sterility 81*, 19–25.

Ferlin, A., Moro, F., Garolla, A. and Foresta, A. (1999) 'Human male infertility and Y chromosome deletions: Role of the AZF-candidate genes DAZ, RBM and DFFRY.' *Human Reproduction 14*, 1710–1716.

Finch, J. and Mason, J. (1993) *Negotiating Family Responsibilities*. London and New York: Routledge.

Forrest, J.D. and Singh, S. (1990) 'The sexual and reproductive behavior of American women 1982–1988.' *Family Planning Perspectives 22*, 206–214.

Frederick, T., Thomas, P., Mascola, L., Hsu, H., Rakusan, T., Mapson, C., Weedon, J. and Bertolli, J. (2000) 'Human immunodeficiency virus-infected adolescents: A descriptive study of older children in New York City, Los Angeles County, Massachusetts and Washington D.C.' *Pediatric Infectious Disease Journal 19*, 6, 551–555.

Freeman, M. (1993) 'The new birth right? Identity and the child of the reproductive revolution.' *The International Journal of Children's Rights 4*, 273–297.

Freud, S. (1901–1905) 'Three essays on sexuality and other writings.' In *Freud: The Standard Edition Vol. 7*. Translated by J. Strachey (1953). London: The Hogarth Press.

Frisch, R.E., Gotz Welbergen, A.V., McArthur, J.W., Albright, T., Witschi, J., Bullen, B., Birnholz, J., Reed, R.B. and Hermann, H. (1981) 'Delayed menarche and amenorrhea of college athletes in relation to age of onset of training.' *Journal of the American Medical Association 246*, 1559–1563.

Fuller, B. and Paynter, S. (2004) 'Fundamentals of cryobiology in reproductive medicine.' *Reproductive Biomedicine Online 9*, 680–691.

Gallagher, B., Christmann, K., Fraser, C. and Hodgson, B. (2003) 'International and internet child sexual abuse and exploitation – issues emerging from research.' *Child and Family Law Quarterly 15*, 4, 353–370.

Gangadharan, Y. (2001) 'Two aspects of fertility behaviour in South Africa.' *Economic Development and Cultural Change 50*, 1, 183–200.

Gillet, D., Braekeleer, M., Bellis, G., Durian, I., French Cystic Fibrosis Registry (2002) 'Cystic fibrosis and pregnancy: Report from French data (1980–99).' *British Journal of Obstetrics and Gynaecology 109*, 912–918.

Gillick v. *West Norfolk and Wisbech Area Health Authority*, 1985. All England Reports 402, HL.

Gilljam, M., Antoniou, M., Shin, J., Dupuis, A. and Corey, M. (2000) 'Pregnancy in cystic fibrosis: Fetal and maternal outcome.' *Chest 118*, 85–91.

Giorgi, A. (1989) 'One type of analysis of descriptive data: Procedures involved in following a scientific phenomenological method.' *Methods (A Journal of Human Science) Annual Edition*, 49–61.

Giwercman, A., Bruun, E., Frimodt-Moller, C. and Skakkebaek, N.E. (1989) 'Prevalence of carcinoma in situ and other histopathological abnormalities in testes of men with a history of cryptorchidism.' *Journal of Urology 142*, 998–1002.

Glaser, A.W., Phelan, L., Crawshaw, M., Jagdev, S. and Hale, J.K. (2004) 'Fertility preservation in adolescent males with cancer in the United Kingdom: A survey of practice.' *Archives of Disease in Childhood 89*, 736–737.

Glaser, A.W., Wilkey, O. and Greenberg, M. (2000) 'Sperm and ova conservation: Existing standards of practice in North America.' *Medical and Pediatric Oncology 35*, 114–118.

Glasgow, D. (1980) *The Black Underclass*. London: Jossey Bass.

Goldman, R. and Goldman, J. (1982) *Children's Sexual Thinking*. London: Routledge and Kegan Paul.

Gordon, C. (1996) 'Adolescent decision-making: A broadly based theory.' *Adolescence 31*, 123, 561–584.

Gosden, R.G. and Spears, N. (1997) 'Programmed cell death in the reproductive system.' *British Medical Bulletin 53*, 644–661.

Gosden, R.G., Baird, D.T., Wade, J.C. and Webb, R. (1994) 'Restoration of fertility to oophorectomized sheep by ovarian autografts stored at −196 degrees C.' *Human Reproduction 9*, 597–603.

Gosden, R.G., Wade, J.C., Fraser, H.M., Sandow, J. and Faddy, M.J. (1997) 'Impact of congenital or experimental hypogonadotrophism on the radiation sensitivity of the mouse ovary.' *Human Reproduction 12*, 2483–2488.

Goss, C.H., Rubenfeld, G.D., Otto, K. and Aitken, M.L. (2003) 'The effect of pregnancy on survival in women with cystic fibrosis.' *Chest 124*, 1460–1468.

Goud, A., Goud, P., Qian, C., Van der Elst, J., Van Maele, G. and Dhont, M. (2000) 'Cryopreservation of human germinal vesicle stage and in vitro matured M II oocytes: Influence of cryopreservation media on the survival, fertilization, and early cleavage divisions.' *Fertility and Sterility 74*, 487–494.

Gougeon, A., Echochard, R. and Thalabard, J.C. (1994) 'Age-related changes of the population of human ovarian follicles: Increase in the disappearance rate of non-growing and early-growing follicles in aging women.' *Biology of Reproduction 50*, 653–663.

Gould, R.L. (1972) 'The phases of adult life: A study of developmental psychology.' *American Journal of Psychiatry 129*, 521–531.

Gray, R.E., Doan, B.D., Schermer, P., Vatter-Fitzgerald, A., Berry, M.P., Jenkin, D. and Doherty, M.A. (1992a) 'Psychologic adaptation of survivors of childhood cancer.' *Cancer 70*, 2713–2721.

Gray, R.E., Doan, B.D., Schermer, P., Vatter-Fitzgerald, A., Berry, M.P., Jenkin, D. and Doherty, M.A. (1992b) 'Surviving childhood cancer: A descriptive approach to understanding the impact of life-threatening illness.' *Psycho-Oncology 1*, 235–245.

Grazi, R.V. and Wolowelsky, J.B. (1995) 'The use of cryopreserved sperm and pre-embryos in contemporary Jewish law and ethics.' *Assisted Reproductive Technology 8*, 53–61.

Green, D. (In press) 'Personal construct theory and paediatric healthcare.' *Clinical Child Psychology and Psychiatry*.

Green, D., Galvin, H. and Horne, B. (2003) 'The psycho-social impact of infertility on young male cancer survivors: A qualitative investigation.' *Psycho-Oncology 12*, 2, 141–152.

Green, D.M., Whitton, J.A., Stovall, M., Mertens, A.C., Donaldson, S.S., Ruymann, F.B., Pendergrass, T.W. and Robison, L.L. (2002) 'Pregnancy outcome of female survivors of childhood cancer: A report from the Childhood Cancer Survivor Study.' *American Journal of Obstetrics and Gynecology 187*, 1070–1080.

Green, D.M., Whitton, J.A., Stovall, M., Mertens, A.C., Donaldson, S.S., Ruymann, F.B., Pendergrass, T.W. and Robison, L.L. (2003) 'Pregnancy outcome of partners of male survivors of childhood cancer: A report from the Childhood Cancer Survivor Study.' *Journal of Clinical Oncology 21*, 4, 716–721.

Greenwell, T.J., Venn, S.N., Creighton, S., Leaver, R.B. and Woodhouse, C.R. (2003) 'Pregnancy after lower urinary tract reconstruction for congenital abnormalities.' *British Journal of Urology International 92*, 7, 773–777.

Greil, A.L. (1991) *Not Yet Pregnant: Infertile Couples in Contemporary America.* New Brunswick, NJ: Rutgers University Press.

Grundy, R., Gosden, R.G., Hewitt, M., Larcher, V., Leiper, A., Spoudeas, H.A., Walker, D. and Wallace, W.H.B. (2001a) 'Fertility preservation for children treated for cancer (1): scientific advances and research dilemmas.' *Archives of Disease in Childhood 84,* 4, 355–359.

Grundy, R., Larcher, V., Gosden, R.G., Hewitt, M., Leiper, A., Spoudeas, H.A., Walker, D. and Wallace, W.H.B. (2001b) 'Fertility preservation for children treated for cancer (2): ethics of consent for gamete storage and experimentation.' *Archives of Disease in Childhood 84,* 4, 360–362.

Gülekli, B., Bulbul, Y., Onvural, A., Yorukoglu, K., Posaci, C., Demir, N. and Erten, O. (1999) 'Accuracy of ovarian reserve tests.' *Human Reproduction 14,* 11, 2822–2826.

Gunaratnam, Y. (1997) 'Culture is not enough: A critique of multiculturalism in palliative care.' In D. Field, J. Hockey and N. Small (eds) *Death, Gender and Ethnicity.* London: Routledge.

Hall, J., Welt, C.K. and Cramer, D.W. (1999) 'Inhibin A and inhibin B reflect ovarian function in assisted reproduction but are less useful at predicting outcome.' *Human Reproduction 14,* 2, 409–415.

Hames, A., Beesley, J. and Nelson, R. (1991) 'Cystic fibrosis: What do patients know and what else would they like to know?' *Respiratory Medicine 85,* 389–392.

Harvey, J., Hobbie, W.L., Shaw, S. and Bottomley, S. (1999) 'Providing quality care in childhood cancer survivorship: Learning from the past, looking to the future.' *Journal of Pediatric Oncology Nursing 16,* 3, 117–125.

Hassold, T., Abruzzo, M., Adkins, K., Griffin, D., Merrill, M., Millie, E., Saker, D., Shen, J. and Zaragoza, M. (1996) 'Human aneuploidy incidence, origin and etiology.' *Environmental and Molecular Mutagenesis 28,* 167–175.

Haugaard, J.J. (2000) 'Defining child sexual abuse.' *American Psychologist 55,* 9, 1036–1039.

Health Protection Agency (2004a) *Epidemiological data – Chlamydia.* Available at www.hpa.org.uk, accessed 19 May 2005.

Health Protection Agency (2004b) *Communicable Diseases Report Weekly 14,* 52, 23 December, available at www.hpa.org.uk, accessed 19 May 2005.

Health Protection Agency (2004c) *Infectious Syphilis; Update to National Data to 2003.* Available at www.hpa.org.uk, accessed 19 May 2005.

Hedley, M. (2000) 'Treating children – whose consent counts?' *Current Paediatrics 10,* 216–218.

Heiman, M.L., Leiblum, S., Cohen Esquilin, S. and Melendez, L. (1998) 'A comparative study of beliefs about "normal" childhood sexual behaviors.' *Child Abuse and Neglect 22,* 4, 289–304.

Heiney, S.P. (1989) 'Adolescents with cancer: Sexual and reproductive issues.' *Cancer Nursing 12,* 2, 95–101.

Heke, S. and Alexander, S. (1995) 'A test-tube too far: Knowledge and attitudes of new reproductive technologies.' Paper presented to the Annual Conference of the Special Group in Health Psychology, British Psychological Society, 6–8 September.

Herek, G.M. and Glunt, E.K. (1998) 'An epidemic of stigma: Public reaction to AIDS.' *American Psychologist 43,* 11, 886–891.

Herek, G.M., Capitanio, J.P. and Widamen, K.F. (2003) 'Stigma, social risk and health policy: Public attitudes towards HIV surveillance policies and the social construct of illness.' *Health Psychology 22,* 5, 533–540.

Herr, H.W., Bar-Chama, N., O'Sullivan, M. and Sogani, P.C. (1998) 'Paternity in men with stage I testis tumours on surveillance.' *Journal of Clinical Oncology 16,* 733–734.

HFEA (Human Fertilisation & Embryology Authority) (1996) 'Reasons for refusing export of semen in Diane Blood case.' Press Release.

HFEA (Human Fertilisation & Embryology Authority) (2001) 'Screening of Patients.' Chairman's Letter Ref CH(01)09.

HFEA (Human Fertilisation & Embryology Authority) (2003) *Code of Practice*. Sixth Edition. London: HFEA.

Hobbie, W.L., Stuber, M., Meeske, K., Wissler, K., Rourke, M.T., Ruccione, K., Hinkle, A. and Kazak, A. (2000) 'Symptoms of post-traumatic stress in young adult survivors of childhood cancer.' *Journal of Clinical Oncology 18*, 24, 4060–4066.

Honaramooz, A., Snedaker, A., Boiani, M., Scholer, H., Dobrinski, I. and Schlatt, S. (2002) 'Sperm from neonatal mammalian testes grafted in mice.' *Nature 418*, 778–781.

Horne, G., Atkinson, A.D., Pease, E.H., Logue, J.P., Brison, D.R. and Lieberman, B.A. (2004) 'Live birth with sperm cryopreserved for 21 years prior to cancer treatment: Case report.' *Human Reproduction 19*, 1448–1449.

Hornor, G. (2004) 'Sexual behavior in children: Normal or not?' *Journal of Pediatric Health Care 18*, 2, 57–64.

Horton, C. (2004) *Working with Children 2004–5*. London: Guardian Books.

Horwitz, S.M., Klerman, L.V., Kuo, H.S. and Jekel, J.F. (1991) 'Intergenerational transmission of school-age parenthood.' *Family Planning Perspectives 23*, 168–172, 177.

House of Commons (2001) *The Royal Liverpool Children's Inquiry*. London: The Stationery Office.

Hovatta, O., Wright, C., Krausz, T., Hardy, K. and Winston, R.M. (1999) 'Human primordial, primary and secondary ovarian follicles in long-term culture: Effect of partial isolation.' *Human Reproduction 14*, 2519–2524.

Howell, S. and Shalet, S. (1998) 'Gonadal damage from chemotherapy and radiotherapy.' *Endocrinology Metabolism Clinics of North America 27*, 927–943.

Howell, S.J. and Shalet, S.M. (2001) 'Testicular function following chemotherapy.' *Human Reproduction Update 7*, 363–369.

Hreinsson, J.G., Otala, M., Fridstrom, M., Borgstrom, B., Rasmussen, C., Lundquist, M., Tuuri, T., Simberg, N., Mikkola, M., Dunkel, L. and Hovatta, O. (2002) 'Follicles are found in the ovaries of adolescent girls with Turner's syndrome.' *Journal of Clinical Endocrinology and Metabolism 87*, 3618–3623.

Hudson, B. (2003) 'From adolescence to young adulthood: The partnership challenge for learning disability services in England.' *Disability & Society 18*, 2, 259–276.

Hull, S.C. and Kass, N.E. (2000) 'Adults with cystic fibrosis and infertility: How has the health care system responded?' *Journal of Andrology 21*, 809–813.

Huntriss, J., Hinkins, M., Oliver, B., Harris, S.E., Beazley, J.C., Rutherford, A.J., Gosden, R.G., Lanzendorf, S.E. and Picton, H.M. (2004) 'Expression of mRNAs for DNA methyltransferases and methyl-CpG-binding proteins in the human female germ line, preimplantation embryos, and embryonic stem cells.' *Molecular Reproduction Development 67*, 323–336.

Hussain, Y., Atkin, K. and Ahmad, W.I.U. (2002) *South Asian Young People and Disability*. Bristol: Policy Press.

Interpol (2005) *Legislation of Interpol Member States on Sexual Offences Against Children*. Available at http://www.interpol.int/Public/Children/SexualAbuse/NationalLaws, accessed 23 May 2005.

Ivey P. (2004) 'Paula is a colon cancer survivor.' www.livestrong.org/livestrong/portal/ep/content, accessed 27 March 2004.

Jacobsen, K.D., Fossa, S.D., Bjoro, T.P., Aass, N., Heilo, A. and Stenwig, A.E. (2002) 'Gonadal function and fertility in patients with bilateral testicular germ cell malignancy.' *European Urology 42*, 229–238.

Jahnukainen, K., Hou, M., Petersen, C., Setchell, B. and Soder, O. (2001) 'Intratesticular transplantation of testicular cells from leukemic rats causes transmission of leukemia.' *Cancer Research 61*, 706–710.

Jin, P., Harris, S.E. and Picton, H.M. (2004) 'The effect of ascorbic acid on ovine preantral follicle development in vitro.' *Reproduction Abstract Series 32*, 22.

Johannessen, M., Carlson, M., Brucefors, A.S. and Hjelte, L. (1998) 'Cystic fibrosis through a female perspective: Psychological issues and information concerning puberty and motherhood.' *Patient Education and Counseling 34*, 115–123.

Johnson, D.S., Russell, L.D. and Griswold, M.D. (2000) 'Advances in spermatogonial stem cell transplantation.' *Reviews of Reproduction 5*, 183–188.

Johnson, M.R.D. (1999) 'Communication in health care: A review of some key issues.' *Nursing Times Research 4*, 1, 18–30.

Jones, S.C. and Hunter, M. (1996) 'The influence of context and discourse on infertility experience.' *Journal of Reproductive and Infant Psychology 14*, 93–111.

Kadan-Lottick, N.S., Robison, L.L., Gurney, J.G., Neglia, J.P., Yasui, Y., Hayashi, R., Hudson, M., Greenberg, M. and Mertens, A.C. (2002) 'Childhood cancer survivors' knowledge about their past diagnosis and treatment: Childhood Cancer Survivor Study.' *Journal of the American Medical Association 287*, 1832–1839.

Kagan-Kreiger, S. (1999) 'The struggle to understand oneself as a woman: Stress, coping and the psychological development of women with Turner syndrome.' EdD. Dissertation, 1998. Canada: OISE/University of Toronto. Source, *Dissertation Abstracts International, A (Humanities and Social Sciences) 59*, 12-A, June, 4368.

Kaplan, E., Schwachman, H., Perlmutter, A.D., Rule, A. and Khaw, K.T. (1968) 'Reproductive failure in males with cystic fibrosis.' *New England Journal of Medicine 279*, 65–69.

Karamesinis, M. (2003) *Hidden Treasure. Thoughts about Living with Turner's Syndrome.* Melbourne: Karamesinis.

Karslen, S. and Nazroo, J.Y. (2002) 'Agency and structure: The impact of ethnic identity and racism on the health of ethnic minority people.' *Sociology of Health and Illness 24*, 1, 1–20.

Katbamna, S., Bhakta, P. and Parker, G. (2000) 'Perceptions of disability and care-giving relationships in South Asian communities.' In W.I.U. Ahmad (ed.) *Ethnicity, Disability and Chronic Illness.* Buckingham: Open University Press.

Katz, A. (2002) *Thwarted Dreams: Young Views from Bradford.* London: Young Voice.

Kelleher, S., Wishart, S.M., Liu, P.Y., Turner, L., Di Pierro, I., Conway, A.J. and Handelsman, D.J. (2001) 'Long-term outcomes of elective human sperm cryostorage.' *Human Reproduction 16*, 2632–2639.

Kempe, C.H. (1978) 'Sexual abuse, another hidden pediatric problem.' *Pediatrics 62*, 382–389.

Kim, S.S., Radford, J., Harris, M., Varley, J., Rutherford, A.J., Lieberman, B., Shalet, S. and Gosden, R. (2001) 'Ovarian tissue harvested from lymphoma patients to preserve fertility may be safe for autotransplantation.' *Human Reproduction 16*, 2056–2060.

King, N. (1994) 'The qualitative research interview.' In C. Cassell and G. Symon (eds) *Qualitative Methods in Organizational Research: A Practical Guide.* London: Sage.

King, N. (1998) 'Template Analysis.' In C. Cassell and G. Symon (eds) *Qualitative Methods and Analysis in Organizational Research.* London: Sage.

Kirby, D. (2001) 'Understanding what works and what doesn't in reducing adolescent sexual risk-taking.' *Family Planning Perspectives 33*, 6, 276–281.

Kirby, D. (2002) 'The impact of schools and school programs upon adolescent sexual behavior.' *Journal of Sex Research 39*, 1, 27–33.

Koeppel, K.M. (1995) 'Sperm banking and patients with cancer: Issues concerning patients and healthcare professionals.' *Cancer Nursing 18*, 4, 306–312.

Kokkonen, J., Vainionpaa, L., Winquist, S. and Lanning, M. (1997) 'Physical and psychosocial outcome for young adults with treated malignancy.' *Pediatric Hematology & Oncology 14*, 223–232.

Koocher, G.P. and O'Malley, J.E. (1981) *The Damocles Syndrome: Psychosocial Consequences of Surviving Childhood Cancer.* New York: McGraw-Hill.

Kopito, L.E., Kosasky, H.J. and Shwachman, H. (1973) 'Water and electrolytes in cervical mucus from patients with cystic fibrosis.' *Fertility and Sterility 24*, 512–516.

Kotloff, R.M., FitzSimmons, S.C. and Fiel, S.B. (1992) 'Fertility and pregnancy in patients with cystic fibrosis.' *Clinics in Chest Medicine 13*, 623–635.

Kun, M., Inglis, J.D. and Sharkey, A. (1993) 'A Y chromosome gene family with RNA-binding protein homology: Candidates for the azoospermia factor for the AZF controlling human spermatogenesis.' *Cell 75*, 1287–1295.

Kwon, J.S. and Case, A.M. (2002) 'Effects of cancer treatment on reproduction and fertility.' *Journal of Obstetrics and Gynaecological Cancer 24*, 8, 619–627.

Lampe, H., Horwich, A., Norman, A., Nicholls, J. and Dearnaley, D.P. (1997) 'Fertility after chemotherapy for testicular germ cell cancers.' *Journal of Clinical Oncology 15*, 239–245.

Langdridge, D., Connolly, K. and Sheeran, P. (2000) 'Reasons for wanting a child: A network analytic study.' *Journal of Reproductive and Infant Psychology 18*, 4, 321–338.

Langeveld, N.E., Ubbink, M.C., Last, B.F., Grootenhuis, M.A., Voute, P.A. and De Haan, R.J. (2003) 'Educational achievement, employment and living situation in long-term young adult survivors of childhood cancer in the Netherlands.' *Psycho-Oncology 12*, 3, 213–225.

Lansdown, G., Waterson, T. and Baum, D. (1996) 'Implementing the UN convention on the rights of the child.' *British Medical Journal 313*, 21–28.

Lansdown, R. (1998) 'Listening to children: Have we gone too far (or not far enough)?' *Journal of the Royal Society of Medicine 91*, 457–461.

Lansky, S.B., List, M.A. and Ritter-Sterr, C. (1986) 'Psychosocial consequences of cure.' *Cancer 58*, 529–533.

Larson, R. and Asmussen, B. (1991) 'Anger, worry and hurt in early adolescence: An enlarging world of negative emotions.' In M.E. Colten and S. Gore (eds) *Adolescent Stress: Causes and Consequences.* New York: Aldine de Gruyter.

Larson, R. and Richards, M. (1994) 'Family emotions: Do young adolescents and their parents experience the same states?' *Journal of Research on Adolescence 4*, 4, 567–583.

Law, I. (1996) *Racism, Ethnicity and Social Policy.* Brighton: Harvester Wheatsheaf.

Leder, D. (ed.) (1992) *The Body in Medical Thought and Practice.* Newhaven: Kluwer Academic Press.

Ledlie, S.W. (1999) 'Diagnosis disclosure by family caregivers to children who have perinatally acquired HIV disease: When the time comes.' *Nursing Research 48*, 3, 141–149.

Ledlie, S.W. (2001) 'The psychosocial issues of children with perinatally acquired HIV disease becoming adolescents: A growing challenge for providers.' *AIDS Patients Care and STDs 15*, 5, 231–236.

Lee, E., Clements, S., Ingham, R. and Stone, N. (2004) *A Matter of Choice? Exploring Reasons for Variations in the Proportions of Under-18 Conceptions that are Terminated.* York: Joseph Rowntree Foundation.

Lee, P.A., Guo, S.S. and Kulin, H.E. (2001) 'Age of puberty: Data from the USA.' *Acta Pathologica Microbiologica et Immunologica Scandinavica (APMIS) 109*, 2, 81–88.

Le Masters, E.E. (1970) *Parents in Modern America: A Sociological Analysis.* Homewood: Dorsey.

Levinson, D.J. and Gooden, W.E. (1985) 'The life cycle.' In N.I. Kaplan and B.J. Sadock (eds) *Comprehensive Textbook of Psychiatry* (Fourth Edition). Baltimore, MD: Williams and Wilkins.

Li, F.P., Fine, W., Jaffe, N., Holmes, G.E. and Holmes, F.F. (1979) 'Offspring of patients treated for cancer in childhood.' *Journal of the National Cancer Institute 62*, 5, 1193–1196.

Liao, L.M. and Boyle, M. (In press) 'Exploring sexuality and relationships.' In M. Cull and S. Creighton (eds) *The AHN Book of Surgery & Dilatation.*

Lipson, M. (1993) 'What do you say to a child with AIDS?' *Hasting Center Report 23*, 2, 6–12.

Lockwood, G., Cooklin, A. and Ramsden, S. (2004) 'Communicating a diagnosis.' In A.H. Balen, S.M. Creighton, M.C. Davies, J. MacDougall and R. Stanhope (eds) *Paediatric and Adolescent Gynaecology.* Cambridge: Cambridge University Press.

Lopez Andreu, J.A., Fernandez, P.J., Ferris i Tortajada, J., Navarro, I., Rodriguez-Ineba, A., Antonio, P., Muro, M.D. and Romeu, A. (2000) 'Persistent altered spermatogenesis in long-term childhood cancer survivors.' *Pediatric Hematology and Oncology 17*, 21–30.

Loughlin, E. (1993) '"Why was I born among mirrors?" Therapeutic dance for teenage girls and women with Turner Syndrome.' *American Journal of Dance Therapy 15*, 2, 107–124.

Loughlin, E. (1998) *The Experience in Dance Movement of Three Individual Women with Turner Syndrome: A Phenomenological Inquiry.* Master Arts Thesis. Melbourne: La Trobe University.

Loughlin, E. (2000) *Same or Different? Creative Interventions and the Response of Adolescent Girls with Turner Syndrome.* Poster, 5th International Turner Symposium – Optimizing Health Care for Turner Patients in the 21st Century, Naples, Italy, March.

Loughlin, E. (2004) *About Fertility, a Semi-structured Group Discussion and Questionnaire with Members of the Victorian Turner's Syndrome Association.* Report.

Loughlin, E. and Werther, G. (2000) 'A phenomenological approach to psychosocial function in Turner syndrome.' In P. Saenger and A. Pasquino (eds) *Optimizing Health Care for Turner Patients in the 21st Century,* Proceedings, 5th International Turner Symposium, Naples, Italy, March. Netherlands: Elsevier Science BV.

Luker, K. (1975) *Taking Chances: Abortion and the Decision Not to Contracept.* Berkeley/Los Angeles: University of California Press.

Luker, K. (1996) *Dubious Conceptions: The Politics of Teenage Pregnancy.* Cambridge, MA: Harvard University Press.

Lyon, A. and Bilton, D. (2002) 'Fertility issues in cystic fibrosis.' *Paediatric Respiratory Reviews 3*, 236–240.

MacDougall, J. (2004) 'The needs of the adolescent patient and her parents in the clinic.' In A.H. Balen, S.M. Creighton, M.C. Davies, J. MacDougall and R. Stanhope (eds) *Paediatric and Adolescent Gynaecology: Management of Developmental Abnormalities and Disorders.* Cambridge: Cambridge University Press.

Mace, D.R., Bannerman, R.H.O. and Burton, J. (1974) 'The teaching of human sexuality in schools for health professionals.' *Public Health Paper 57.* Geneva: World Health Organization.

Macpherson, W. (1999) *The Stephen Lawrence Inquiry: Report of an Inquiry by Sir William Macpherson of Cluny* (Cm 4262-I). London: HMSO.

Madge, S.L. and Carr, S.B. (1999) 'Reproductive health in males with cystic fibrosis: Knowledge, attitudes and experience of patients and parents.' (Letter) *Pediatric Pulmonology 27*, 293.

Mahlstedt, P.P. (1985) 'The psychological components of infertility.' *Fertility and Sterility 43*, 335–346.

Malus, M., LaChance, P., Lamy, L., Macaulay, A. and Vanasse, M. (1987) 'Priorities in adolescent health care: A teenager's view-point.' *Journal of Family Practice 25*, 159–162.

Mantzoros, C.S., Flier, J.S. and Rogol, A.D. (1997) 'A longitudinal assessment of hormonal and physical alterations during normal puberty in boys. V. Rising leptin levels may signal the onset of puberty.' *Journal of Clinical Endocrinology and Metabolism 82*, 1066–1070.

Marsden, D. and Hacker, N. (2003) 'Fertility effects of cancer treatment.' *Australian Family Physician 32*, 1/2, 9–13.

Marsiglio, W. (1993) 'Adolescent males' orientation toward paternity and contraception.' *Family Planning Perspectives 25*, 1, 22–31.

Masala, A., Faedda, R., Alagna, S., Satta, A., Chiarelli, G., Rovasio, P., Ivaldi, R., Taras, M.S., Lai, E. and Bartoli, E. (1997) 'Use of testosterone to prevent cyclophosphamide-induced azoospermia.' *Annals of Internal Medicine 126*, 292–295.

Mason, D. (2000) *Race and Ethnicity in Modern Britain.* Oxford: Oxford University Press.

May, B., Boyle, M. and Grant, D. (1996) 'A comparative study of sexual experiences.' *Journal of Health Psychology 1*, 4, 479–492.

McCabe, M.P. and Killackey, E.J. (2004) 'Sexual decision making in young women.' *Sexual and Relationship Therapy 19*, 1, 15–27.

McCall Smith, J. (2004) 'Legal issues: UK perspective.' In H. Wallace and D. Green (eds) *Late Effects of Childhood Cancer.* London: Arnold.

McCallum, T.J., Milunsky, J.M., Cunningham, D.L., Harris, D.H. and Maher, T.A. (2000) 'Fertility in men with CF: An update on current surgical practices and outcomes.' *Chest 118*, 1059–1062.

McLachlan, R.I., Robertson, D.M., Healy, D.L., de Kretser, D.M. and Burger, H.G. (1986) 'Plasma inhibin levels during gonadotropin-induced ovarian hyperstimulation for IVF: A new index of follicular function?' *Lancet 1*, 8492, 1233–1234.

Meirow, D. (2000) 'Reproduction post-chemotherapy in young cancer patients.' *Molecular and Cellular Endocrinology 169*, 123–131.

Meirow, D. and Nugent, D. (2001) 'The effects of radiotherapy and chemotherapy on female reproduction.' *Human Reproduction Update 7*, 535–543.

Meirow, D., Fasouliotis, S.J., Nugent, D., Schenker, J.G., Gosden, R.G. and Rutherford, A.J. (1999a) 'A laparoscopic technique for obtaining ovarian cortical biopsy specimens for fertility conservation in patients with cancer.' *Fertility and Sterility 71*, 948–951.

Meirow, D., Lewis, H., Nugent, D. and Epstein, M. (1999b) 'Subclinical depletion of primordial follicular reserve in mice treated with cyclophosphamide: Clinical importance and proposed accurate investigative tool.' *Human Reproduction 14*, 1903–1907.

Meistrich, M.L. (1993) 'Effects of chemotherapy and radiotherapy on spermatogenesis.' *European Urology 23*, 136–142.

Meistrich, M.L. and Shetty, G. (2003) 'Supression of testosterone stimulates recovery of spermatogenesis after cancer treatment.' *International Journal of Andrology 26*, 141–146.

Melton, L. (2001) 'New perspectives on the management of intersex.' *Lancet 357*, 2110.

Merke, D.P., Fields, J.D., Keil, M.F., Vaituzis, A.C., Chrousos, G.P. and Giedd, J.N. (2003) 'Children with classic Congenital Adrenal Hyperplasia have decreased amygdala volume:

potential prenatal and postnatal hormonal effects.' *Journal of Clinical Endocrinology & Metabolism 88*, 4, 1760–1765.

Merrick, E.N. (1995) 'Adolescent childbearing as career "choice": Perspectives from an ecological context.' *Journal of Counseling and Development 73*, 288–295.

Mertineit, C., Yoder, J.A., Taketo, T., Laird, D.W., Trasler, J.M. and Bestor, T.H. (1998) 'Sex-specific exons control DNA methyltransferase in mammalian germ cells.' *Development 125*, 889–897.

Meseguer, M., Garrido, N., Remohi, J., Pellicer, A., Simon, C., Martínez-Jabaloyas, J.M. and Gil-Salom, M. (2003) 'Testicular sperm extraction (TESE) and ICSI in patients with permanent azoospermia after chemotherapy.' *Human Reproduction 18*, 1281–1285.

Meyer-Bahlburg, H.F.L. (2001) 'Gender and sexuality in classic congenital adrenal hyperplasia.' *Endocrinology and Metabolism Clinics of North America 30*, 155–171, VIII.

Miall, C.E. (1985) 'Perceptions of informal sanctioning and the stigma of involuntary childlessness.' *Deviant Behavior 6*, 383–403.

Michelmore, K.F., Ong, K., Mason, S., Bennett, S., Perry, L., Vessey, M.P., Balen, A.H. and Dunger, D.B. (2001) 'Clinical features in women with polycystic ovaries: Relationships to insulin sensitivity, insulin gene *VNTR* and birth weight.' *Clinical Endocrinology 55*, 439–446.

Miller, K.A., Elkind-Hirsch, K., Levy, B., Graubert, M.D., Ross, S.J. and Scott, R.T., Jr. (2004) 'Pregnancy after cryopreservation of donor oocytes and preimplantation genetic diagnosis of embryos in a patient with ovarian failure.' *Fertility and Sterility 82*, 211–214.

Miller, W.B. (1995) 'Childbearing motivation and its measurement.' *Journal of Biosocial Sciences 27*, 473–487.

Minto, C., Creighton, S. and Woodhouse, C. (2001) 'Long term sexual function in intersex conditions with ambiguous genitalia.' *Journal of Pediatric and Adolescent Gynecology 14*, 141–142.

Minto, C.L., Liao, L.-M., Woodhouse, C.R.J., Ransley, P.G. and Creighton, S.M. (2003) 'The effect of clitoral surgery on sexual outcome in individuals who have intersex conditions with ambiguous genitalia: A cross-sectional study.' *Lancet 361*, 1252–1257.

Mir, G. and Nocon, A. (2002) 'Partnership, advocacy and independence: Service principles and the empowerment of minority ethnic people.' *Journal of Learning Disabilities 6*, 2, 153–162.

Mir, G. and Tovey, P. (2003) 'Asian carers' experience of medical and social care: The case of cerebral palsy.' *British Journal of Social Work 33*, 465–479.

Mischler, E.H., Wilfond, B.S., Fost, N., Laxova, A., Reiser, C. and Sauer, C.M. (1998) 'Cystic fibrosis newborn screening: Impact on reproductive behavior and implications for genetic counseling.' *Pediatrics 102*, 44–52.

Modood, T., Betthould, R. and Lakey, J. (1997) *Ethnic Minorities in Britain.* London: Social Policy Studies Institute.

Money, J., Schwartz, M. and Lewis, V.G. (1984) 'Adult eretosexual status and fetal hormonal masculinization and demasculinization: 46 XX Congenital Virilizing Adrenal Hyperplasia and 46 XY Androgen Insensitivity Syndrome compared.' *Psychoneuroendocrinology 9*, 405–414.

Morell, C. (2000) 'Saying no: Women's experiences with reproductive refusal.' *Feminism in Psychology 10*, 3, 313–322.

Morgan, J.F., Murphy, H., Lacey, J.H. and Conway, G.S. (2005) 'Long term psychological outcome for women with Congenital Adrenal Hyperplasia: Cross sectional survey.' *British Medical Journal 330*, 340–341.

Morita, Y. and Tilly, J.L. (2000) 'Sphingolipid regulation of female gonadal cell apoptosis.' *Annals of the New York Academy of Science 905*, 209–220.

Morita, Y., Perez, G.I., Paris, F., Miranda, S.R., Ehleiter, D., Haimovitz-Friedman, A., Fuks, Z., Xie, Z., Reed, J.C., Schuchman, E.H., Kolesnick, R.N. and Tilly, J.L. (2000) 'Oocyte apoptosis is suppressed by disruption of the acid sphingomyelinase gene or by sphingosine-1-phosphate therapy.' *Nature Medicine 6*, 1109–1114.

Morris, J. (2002) 'Moving into adulthood: Young disabled people moving into adulthood.' JRF Findings Ref 512. York: Joseph Rowntree Foundation. http://www.jrf.org.uk/knowledge/findings/foundations/512.asp, accessed on 21 July 2005.

Morrow, V. (1998) *Understanding Families: Children's Perspectives*. London: National Children's Bureau.

Morse, C. (2000) 'Reproduction: A critical analysis.' In J.M. Ussher *Women's Health: Contemporary International Perspectives*. Leicester: BPS Books.

Mortimer, D. (1994) *Practical Laboratory Andrology*. Oxford: Oxford University Press.

Moustakas, C. (1994) *Phenomenological Research Methods*. Thousand Oaks, CA: Sage.

Mullen, S.F., Agca, Y., Broermann, D.C., Jenkins, C.L., Johnson, C.A. and Critser, J.K. (2004) 'The effect of osmotic stress on the metaphase II spindle of human oocytes, and the relevance to cryopreservation.' *Human Reproduction 19*, 1148–1154.

Multi-disciplinary Working Group (2003) 'A strategy for fertility services for survivors of childhood cancer.' *Human Fertility 6*, 2, A1–A40.

Murphy, D.A., Durako, S.J., Moscicki, A.B., Vermund, S.H., Ma, Y., Schwarz, D.F., Muenz, L.R., Adolescent Medicines HIV/AIDS Research Network (2001) 'No change in health risk behaviors over time among HIV infected adolescents in care: Role of psychological distress.' *Journal of Adolescent Health 29*, 3, 57–63.

Musick, J.S. (1993) *Young, Poor, and Pregnant: The Psychology of Teenage Motherhood*. New Haven, CT: Yale University Press.

National Institute for Clinical Excellence (NICE) (2004) *Fertility: Assessment and Treatment for People with Fertility Problems*. Clinical Guideline, Developed by National Collaborating Centre for Women's and Children's Health February 2004. Accessed at http://www.nice.org.uk.

Nazroo, J.Y. (1997) 'The health of Britain's ethnic minorities – findings from a national survey.' *The Fourth National Survey of Ethnic Minorities*. London: Policy Studies Institute.

Neal, A.G., Groat, H.T. and Wicks, J.W. (1989) 'Attitudes about having children: A study of 600 couples in the early years of marriage.' *Journal of Marriage and the Family 51*, 313–328.

Netherwood, P.E. (1998) 'A study of the psychological impact of infertility on men and of the process of adjustment to diagnosis and treatment options.' Unpublished thesis (D.Clin.Psycol.), University of Leeds.

Netto, G., Gaag, S., Thanki, M., Bondi, L. and Munro, M. (2001) *A Suitable Space: Improving Counselling Services for Asian People*. Joseph Rowntree Foundation: Policy Press.

Neville, K. (1998) 'The relationships among uncertainty, social support and psychological distress in adolescents recently diagnosed with cancer.' *Journal of Pediatric Oncology Nursing 15*, 37–46.

Newton, H., Aubard, Y., Rutherford, A.J., Sharma, V. and Gosden, R.G. (1996) 'Low temperature storage and grafting of human ovarian tissue.' *Human Reproduction 11*, 1487–1491.

Newton, H., Picton, H.M. and Gosden, R.G. (1999) 'In vitro growth of preantral follicles isolated from frozen/thawed ovine tissue.' *Journal of Reproduction and Fertility 115*, 141–150.

Nixon, G.M., Glazner, J.A., Martin, J.M. and Sawyer, S.M. (2003) 'Female sexual health care in cystic fibrosis.' *Archives of Disease in Childhood 88*, 265–266.

Nizalova, O. (2000) 'Economic and social consequences of maternal protection: A cross-country analysis.' http://www.gdnet.org/pdf/948_Nizalova_paper2000-1.pdf.

Nolan, T., Desmond, K., Herlich, R. and Hardy, S. (1986) 'Knowledge of cystic fibrosis in patients and their parents.' *Pediatrics 77*, 229–235.

Nugent, D., Newton, H., Gallivan, L. and Gosden, R.G. (1998) 'Protective effect of vitamin E on ischaemia-reperfusion injury in ovarian grafts.' *Journal of Reproduction and Fertility 114*, 341–346.

O'Brien, M.J., Pendola, J.K. and Eppig, J.J. (2003) 'A revised protocol for in vitro development of mouse oocytes from primordial follicles dramatically improves their developmental competence.' *Biology of Reproduction 68*, 1682–1686.

O'Connell, H.E., Hutson, J.M., Anderson, C.R. and Plenter, R.J. (1998) 'Anatomical relationship between urethra and clitoris.' *Journal of Urology 159*, 1892–1897.

Odegaard, I., Stray-Pederen, B., Hallberg, K., Haanes, O.C. and Storrosten, O.T. (2002) 'Prevalence and outcome of pregnancies in Norwegian and Swedish women with CF.' *Acta Obstetricia Gynecologica Scandinavica 81*, 693–697.

Oeffinger, K.C., Eshelman, D., Tomlinson, G.E. and Buchanan, G.R. (1998) 'Programs for adult survivors of childhood cancer.' *Journal of Clinical Oncology 16*, 8, 2864–2867.

Ogilvy-Stuart, A.L. and Brain, C.E. (2004) 'Early assessment of ambiguous genitalia.' *Archives of Disease in Childhood 89*, 401–407.

Oktay, K. and Karlikaya, G. (2000) 'Ovarian function after transplantation of frozen, banked, autologous ovarian tissue.' *New England Journal of Medicine 342*, 1919.

Oktay, K. and Yih, M. (2002) 'Preliminary experience with orthotopic and heterotopic transplantation of ovarian cortical strips.' *Seminars in Reproductive Medicine 20*, 63–74.

Oktay, K., Buyuk, E., Veeck, L., Zaninovic, N., Xu, K., Takeuchi, T., Opsahl, M. and Rosenwaks, Z. (2004) 'Embryo development after heterotopic transplantation of cryopreserved ovarian tissue.' *Lancet 363*, 837–840.

Olechnowicz, J.Q., Eder, M., Simon, C., Zyzanski, S. and Kodish, E. (2002) 'Assent observed: Children's involvement in leukemia treatment and research discussions.' *Pediatrics 109*, 806–814.

Oliver, M. (1996) *Understanding Disability: From Theory to Practice.* Basingstoke: Macmillan.

Ondrusek, N., Abramovitch, R., Pencharz, P. and Koren, G. (1998) 'Empirical examination of the ability of children to consent to clinical research.' *Journal of Medical Ethics 24*, 158–165.

Orr, D.P., Hoffmans, M.A. and Bennetts, G. (1984) 'Adolescents with cancer report their psychosocial needs.' *Journal of Psychosocial Oncology 2*, 2, 47–59.

Orten, J.L. and Orten, J.D. (1994) 'Women with Turner's Syndrome: Helping them reach their full potential.' *Disability & Society 9*, 2, 239–248.

Pacey, A.A. (2003) 'Sperm you can bank on.' *British Medical Journal 327*, 1354.

Palermo, G., Joris, H., Derde, M.P., Camus, M., Devroe, Y.P. and Van Steirtegehm, A.C. (1995) 'Intracytoplasmic sperm injection: A novel treatment for all forms of male factor infertility.' *Fertility and Sterility 63*, 1231–1240.

Papastergiadis, N. (1982) *Dialogues in the Diasporas: Essays and Conversations on Cultural Identity.* London/New York: Rivers Oram Press.

Parekh, B. (2000) *Rethinking Multi-Culturalism: Cultural Diversity and Political Theory.* Basingstoke: Palgrave.

Parkes, C.M. and Markus, A. (eds) (1998) *Coping with Loss.* London: BMJ Books.

Parks, J.E., Lee, D.R., Huang, S. and Kaproth, M.T. (2003) 'Prospects for spermatogenesis *in vitro*.' *Theriogenology 59*, 73–86.

Patton, G.A. (1999) 'Briefing paper for the National Public Health Partnership.' National Public Health Partnership, Melbourne: Centre for Adolescent Health, Royal Children's Hospital.

Payne, J. (2004) 'The impact of a reduced fertility rate on women's health.' *BMC Women's Health 4* (Suppl.1), S11.

Pearlin, L.I. (1989) 'The sociological study of stress.' *Journal of Health and Social Behavior 30*, 241–256.

Pendley, J.S., Dahlquist, L.M. and Dreyer, Z. (1997) 'Body image and psychosocial adjustment in adolescent cancer survivors.' *Journal of Pediatric Psychology 22*, 1, 29–44.

Pereyra Pacheco, B., Mendez Ribas, J.M., Milone, G., Fernandez, I., Kvicala, R., Mila, T., Di Noto, A., Contreras Ortiz, O. and Pavlovsky, S. (2001) 'Use of GnRH analogs for functional protection of the ovary and preservation of fertility during cancer treatment in adolescents: A preliminary report.' *Gynecological Oncology 81*, 391–397.

Pfeffer, N. and Woollett, A. (1983) *The Experience of Infertility*. London: Virago.

Phelan, M. and Parkman, S. (1995) 'How to work with an interpreter.' *British Medical Journal 311*, 555–557.

Phelan, P.D., Allen, J.L. and Barnes, G.L. (1979) 'Improved survival of patients with cystic fibrosis.' *Medical Journal of Australia 1*, 261–263.

PHLS Aids Centre and the Scottish Centre for Infection and Environmental Health (2002) *Aids/HIV Quarterly Surveillance Tables: Cumulative UK Data to End December 2001*. London: Public Health Laboratory Service.

Picton, H.M. (2002) 'Oocyte maturation in vitro.' *Current Opinion in Obstetrics and Gynecology 14*, 295–302.

Picton, H.M., Briggs, D. and Gosden, R.G. (1998) 'The molecular basis of oocyte growth and development.' *Molecular and Cellular Endocrinology 145*, 27–37.

Picton, H.M., Danfour, M.A., Harris, S.E., Chambers, E.L. and Huntriss, J. (2003) 'Growth and maturation of oocytes in vitro.' *Reproduction Supplement 61*, 445–462.

Picton, H.M., Gosden, R.G. and Leibo, S.P. (2003) 'Cryopreservation of oocytes and ovarian tissue.' In E. Vayena, P. Rowe and P. Griffin (eds) *Current Practices and Controversies on Assisted Reproduction*. Geneva: World Health Organization.

Picton, H.M., Harris, S.E. and Chambers, E.L. (2004) 'Prospects for follicle culture.' In T. Tulandi and R.G. Gosden (eds) *Preservation of Fertility*. London: Parthenon Publishing Group.

Picton, H.M., Kim, S.S. and Gosden, R.G. (2000) 'Cryopreservation of gonadal tissue and cells.' *British Medical Bulletin 56*, 603–615.

Pleck, J., Sonnenstein, F. and Leighton, C. (1993) 'Masculinity ideology: Its impact on adolescent males' heterosexual relationships.' *Journal of Social Issues 49*, 11–19.

Polson, D.W., Adams, J., Wadsworth, J. and Franks, S. (1988) 'Polycystic ovaries – a common finding in normal women.' *Lancet 1*, 8590, 870–872.

Porcu, E., Fabbri, R., Damiano, G., Giunchi, S., Fratto, R., Ciotti, P.M., Venturoli, S. and Flamigni, C. (2000) 'Clinical experience and applications of oocyte cryopreservation.' *Molecular and Cellular Endocrinology 169*, 33–37.

Punch, S. (2003) 'Childhoods in the majority world: Miniature adults or tribal children?' *Sociology 37*, 2, 277–298.

Puukko, L.R., Sammallahti, P.R., Slimes, M.A. and Aalberg, V.A. (1997) 'Childhood leukaemia and body image: Interview reveals impairment not found with a questionnaire.' *Journal of Clinical Psychology 53*, 2, 133–137.

Quinlivan, J.A. and Evans, S.F. (2000) 'The impact of domestic violence in teenage pregnancy – a prospective cohort study.' *Journal of Pediatrics and Adolescent Gynecology 14*, 17–23.

Qureshi, H. and Walker, A. (1989) *The Caring Relationship*. Basingstoke: Macmillan.

Qureshi, T., Berridge, D. and Wenman, H. (2000) *Where to Turn? Family Support for South Asian Communities: A Case Study*. London: Joseph Rowntree Foundation.

Radford, J., Lieberman, B.A., Brison, D.R., Smith, A.R., Critchlow, J.D., Russell, S.A., Watson, A.J., Clayton, J.A., Harris, M., Gosden, R.G. and Shalet, S.M. (2001) 'Orthotopic reimplantation of cryopreserved ovarian cortical strips after high-dose chemotherapy for Hodgkin's lymphoma.' *Lancet 357*, 1172–1175.

Radford, J., Shalet, S. and Lieberman, B. (1999) 'Fertility after treatment for cancer: Questions remain over ways of preserving ovarian and testicular tissue.' *British Medical Journal 319*, 935–936.

Ragni, G., Caccamo, A.M., Dalla Serra, A. and Guercilena, S. (1990) 'Computerized slow-stage freezing of semen from men with testicular tumors of Hodgkin's disease preserves sperm better than standard vapor freezing.' *Fertility and Sterility 53*, 1072–1075.

Rainey, D., Stevens-Simon, C. and Kaplan, D.W. (1993) 'Self-perception of infertility among female adolescents.' *American Journal of Diseases of Children 147*, 1053–1056.

Rajkowha, M., Glass, M.R., Rutherford, A.J., Michelmore, K. and Balen, A.H. (2000) 'Polycystic Ovary Syndrome: A risk factor for cardiovascular disease?' *British Journal of Obstetrics and Gynaecology 107*, 11–18.

Raphael-Leff, J. (1991) *Psychological Processes of Childbearing*. London: Chapman and Hall.

Reich, W. (1968) *The Function of the Orgasm*. London: Panther.

Reik, W. and Walter, J. (2001) 'Genomic imprinting: Parental influence on the genome.' *Nature Reviews Genetics 2*, 21–32.

Relander, T., Cavallin-Stahl, E., Garwicz, S., Olsson, A.M. and Willwn, M. (2000) 'Gonadal and sexual function in men treated for childhood cancer.' *Medical and Pediatric Oncology 35*, 52–63.

Rickert, V., Hassed, S., Hendon, A. and Cunniff, C. (1996) 'The effects of peer ridicule on depression and self-image among adolescent females with Turner syndrome.' *Journal of Adolescent Health 19*, 1, 34–38.

Rindfuss, R.R., Morgan, S.P. and Offutt, K. (1996) 'Education and the changing age pattern of American fertility 1963–1989.' *Demography 33*, 3, 277–290.

Ritchie, J. and Spencer, J. (1994) 'Qualitative data analysis for applied policy research.' In A. Bryman and R.G. Burgess (eds) *Analysing Qualitative Data*. London: Routledge.

Robbins, W.A., Meistrich, M., Moore, D., Hagemeister, F.B., Weier, H.U., Cassel, M.J., Wilson, G., Eskenazi, B. and Wyrobek, A.J. (1997) 'Chemotherapy induces transient sex chromosomal and autosomal aneuploidy in human sperm.' *Nature Genetics 16*, 74–78.

Roberts, C., Piper, L., Denny, J. and Cuddeback, G. (1997) 'A support group intervention to facilitate young adults' adjustment to cancer.' *Health and Social Work 22*, 2, 133–141.

Roberts, C.S., Turney, M.E. and Knowles, A.M. (1998) 'Psychosocial issues of adolescents with cancer.' *Social Work in Health Care 27*, 4, 3–18.

Roberts, H. and Sachdev, D. (1996) *Young People's Social Attitudes. Having Their Say: The Views of 12–19 Year Olds*. Barkingside: Barnardos.

Robinson, K., Price, J., Thompson, C. and Schmalzried, H. (1998) 'Rural junior school students' risk factors for and perceptions of teenage parenthood.' *Journal of School Health 68*, 334–343.

Robinson, M. (2001) *Communication and Health in a Multi-Ethnic Society*. Bristol: Policy Press.

Robson, C. (1998) *Real World Research*. Oxford: Blackwell.

Rodriquez, C. and Gore, N.B. (1995) 'Perceptions of pregnant/parenting teens: Reframing issues for an integrated approach to pregnancy problems.' *Adolescence 30*, 685–706.

Rofeim, O. and Gilbert, B.R. (2004) 'Normal semen parameters in cancer patients presenting for cryopreservation before gonadotoxic therapy.' *Fertility and Sterility 82*, 505–506.

Rogstad, K.E., Ahmed-Jushuf, I.H. and Robinson, A.J. (2002) 'Standards for comprehensive sexual health services for young people under 25 years.' *International Journal of STD and AIDS 13*, 420–424.

Rosenlund, B., Sjoblam, P., Dimitrakopoulos, A. and Hillensjo, T. (1997) 'Epididymal and testicular sperm injection in the treatment of obstructive azospermia.' *Acta Obstetricia Gynecologica Scandinavica 75*, 135–139.

Ross, J.W. and Scarvalone, S.A. (1982) 'Facilitating the pediatric cancer patient's return to school.' *Social Work 27*, 3, 256–261.

Rotheram-Borus, M.J., Weiss, R., Alber, S. and Lester, P. (2005) 'Adolescent adjustment before and after HIV-related parental death.' *Journal of Consulting and Clinical Psychology 73*, 2, 221–228.

Rowland, J.H. (1990) 'Developmental stage and adaptation: Child and adolescent model.' In J.C. Holland and J.H. Rowland (eds) *Handbook of Psychooncology*. New York, NY: Oxford University Press.

Royal College of Physicians (1996) *Guidelines on the Practice of Ethics Committees in Medical Research Involving Human Subjects*. London: Royal College of Physicians.

Rushforth, H. (1999) 'Practitioner review: Communicating with hospitalised children: Review and application of research pertaining to children's understanding of health and illness.' *Journal of Child Psychology and Psychiatry 40*, 5, 683–691.

Ryan, G. (2000) 'Childhood sexuality: A decade of study. Part 1 – research and curriculum development.' *Child Abuse and Neglect 24*, 1, 33–48.

Ryan, G., Miyoshi, T. and Krugman, R. (1988) 'Early childhood experience of professionals working in child abuse.' 17th Annual Symposium on Child Abuse and Neglect, Keystone, Colorado.

Saenger, P., Albertsson Wikland, K., Conway, G., Davenport, M., Gravholt, C., Hintz, R., Hovatta, O., Hultcrantz, M., Landin-Wilhelmsen, K., Lin, A., Lippe, B., Pasquino, A., Ranke, M., Rosenfeld, R. and Silberbach, M. (2001) 'Recommendations for the diagnosis and management of Turner syndrome.' *Journal of Clinical Endocrinology & Metabolism 86*, 7, 3061–3069.

Salle, B., Demirci, B., Franck, M., Berthollet, C. and Lornage, J. (2003) 'Long-term follow-up of cryopreserved hemi-ovary autografts in ewes: Pregnancies, births, and histologic assessment.' *Fertility and Sterility 80*, 172–177.

Sawyer, S.M. (2000) 'Reproductive and sexual health.' In M.E. Hodson and D.M. Geddes (eds) *Cystic Fibrosis*. Second Edition. London: Arnold Publishers.

Sawyer, S.M. and Glazner, J. (2004) 'What follows neonatal screening? An evaluation of an assessment and education program for parents of newly diagnosed infants with cystic fibrosis.' *Pediatrics 114*, 411–416.

Sawyer, S.M., Farrant, B., Cerritelli, B. and Wilson, J. (2005) 'A survey of sexual and reproductive health in men with cystic fibrosis: New challenges for adolescent and adult services.' *Thorax 60*, 326–330.

Sawyer, S.M., Phelan, P.D. and Bowes, G. (1995) 'Reproductive health in young women with cystic fibrosis: Knowledge, attitudes and behaviour.' *Journal of Adolescent Health 17*, 46–50.

Sawyer, S.M., Rosier, M.J., Phelan, P.D. and Bowes, G. (1995) 'The self-image of adolescents with cystic fibrosis.' *Journal of Adolescent Health 16*, 204–208.

Sawyer, S.M., Tully, M.A. and Colin, A.A. (2001) 'Reproductive and sexual health in men with cystic fibrosis: A case for health professional education and training.' *Journal of Adolescent Health 28*, 36–40.

Sawyer, S.M., Tully, M.A., Dovey, M.E. and Colin, A.A. (1998) 'Reproductive health in males with CF: Knowledge, attitudes and experiences of patients and parents.' *Pediatric Pulmonology 25*, 226–230.

Scannapieco, M. and Jackson, S. (1996) 'The African American response to family preservation.' *Social Work 4*, 12, 190–196.

Schechter, N.L., Berrien, F.B. and Katz, S.M. (1988) 'PCA for adolescents in sickle-cell crisis.' *American Journal of Nursing 88*, 5, 719, 721–722.

Schlatt, S. (2002) 'Germ cell transplantation.' *Molecular and Cellular Endocrinology 186*, 163–167.

Schmid, J., Kirchengast, S., Vytiska-Binsorfer, E. and Huber, J. (2004) 'Infertility caused by PCOS-health related quality of life among Austrian and Moslem immigrant women in Austria.' *Human Reproduction 19*, 10, 2251–2257.

Schover, L.R. (1997) *Sexuality and Fertility after Cancer.* New York: John Wiley and Sons.

Schover, L.R. (1999) 'Psychosocial aspects of infertility and decisions about reproduction in young cancer survivors: A review.' *Medical and Pediatric Oncology 33*, 1, 53–59.

Schover, L.R., Brey, K., Lichtin, A., Lipshultz, L.I. and Sima, J. (2002) 'Oncologists' attitudes and practices regarding banking sperm before cancer treatment.' *Journal of Clinical Oncology 20*, 7, 1 April, 1890–1897.

Schover, L.R., Rybicki, L.A., Martin, B.A. and Bringelsen, K.A. (1999) 'Having children after cancer: A pilot survey of survivors' attitudes and experiences.' *Cancer 86*, 4, 667–709.

Schroder, C.P., Timmer-Bosscha, H., Wijchman, J.G., de Leij, L.F., Hollema, H., Heineman, M.J. and de Vries, E.G. (2004) 'An in vitro model for purging of tumour cells from ovarian tissue.' *Human Reproduction 19*, 1069–1075.

Schubotz, D., Rolston, B. and Simpson, A. (2004) 'Sexual behaviour of young people in Northern Ireland: First sexual experience.' *Critical Public Health 14*, 2, 177–190.

Schultz Adams, H. (2003) 'Young adults with cancer.' *Cure, Summer Issue 2*, 2, 36–41.

Scotet, V., de Braekeleer, M., Roussey, M., Rault, G., Parent, P. and Dagome, M. (2000) 'Neonatal screening for cystic fibrosis in Brittany, France: Assessment of 10 years' experience and impact on prenatal diagnosis.' *Lancet 356*, 789–794.

Sharara, F.I. and McClamrock, H.D. (1999) 'The effect of aging on ovarian volume measurements in infertile women.' *Obstetrics & Gynecology 94*, 1, 57–60.

Sharp, M.C., Struss, R.P. and Lorch, S.C. (1992) 'Communicating medical bad news: Parents' experiences and preferences.' *Journal of Pediatrics 121*, 539–546.

Shaw, J. and Trounson, A.O. (1997) 'Ovarian banking for cancer patients – oncological implications in the replacement of ovarian tissue.' *Human Reproduction 12*, 403–405.

Shaw, J.M., Oranratnachai, A. and Trounson, A.O. (2000) 'Fundamental cryobiology of mammalian oocytes and ovarian tissue.' *Theriogenology 53*, 59–72.

Sherman, B.F., Bonanno, G.A., Wiener, L.S. and Battles, H.B. (2000) 'When children tell their friends they have AIDS: Possible consequences for psychological well-being and disease progression.' *Psychosomatic Medicine 62*, 238–247.

Sherman, J.K. (1963) 'Improved methods of preservation of human spermatozoa by freezing and freeze-drying.' *Fertility and Sterility 14*, 49–64.

Sinason, V. (1992) *Mental Handicap and the Human Condition: New Approaches from the Tavistock.* London: Free Association Press.

Singh, K.L., Davies, M. and Chatterjee, R. (2005) 'Fertility in female cancer survivors: Pathophysiology, preservation and the role of ovarian reserve testing.' *Human Reproductive Update 11,* 1, 69–89.

Skakkebaek, N.E., Giwercman, A. and de Krester, D. (1994) 'Pathogenesis and management of male infertility.' *Lancet 343,* 1473–1478.

Slijper, F., van Teunenbroek, A., de Muinck Keizer-Schrama, S. and Sas, T. (1998) Abstract. 'A daughter with Turner's syndrome: An impact on parents.' (Dutch.) *Nederlands Tijdschrift voor Geneeskunde 142,* 39, 2150–2158.

Smaje, C. and Field, D. (1997) 'Absent minorities? Ethnicity and the use of palliative care services.' In D. Field, J. Hockey and N. Small (eds) *Death, Gender and Ethnicity.* London: Routledge.

Smallwood, S. and Jefferies, J. (2003) 'Family building intentions in England and Wales: Trends, outcomes and interpretations.' *Population Trends 112,* 15–28.

Smith, G.D. and Silva, E.S.C.A. (2004) 'Developmental consequences of cryopreservation of mammalian oocytes and embryos.' *Reproductive Biomedicine Online 9,* 171–178.

Sobsey, R. (1992) 'What we know about abuse and disabilities.' *NRCCSA News Nov/Dec.* Huntsville: National Resource Center on Child Sexual Abuse.

Social Services Inspectorate (SSI) (2000) *A Jigsaw of Services: Inspection of Services to Support Disabled Adults in their Parenting Role.* CI(2000)6. London: Department of Health.

Stacy Nicholson, H. and Byrne, J. (1993) 'Fertility and pregnancy after treatment for cancer during childhood or adolescence.' *Cancer 71,* 10, 3392–3399.

Stead, M.L., Fallowfield, L., Brown, J.M. and Selby, P. (2001) 'Communication about sexual problems and sexual concerns in ovarian cancer: Qualitative study.' *British Medical Journal 323,* 835–837.

Stephen, E.H. and Chandra, A. (1998) 'Updated projections of infertility in the United States: 1995–2025.' *Fertility and Sterility 70,* 30–34.

Stern, R.C., Doershuck, C.F. and Drumm, M. (1995) '3849+10kb C-T mutation and disease severity in cystic fibrosis.' *Lancet 346,* 274–276.

Stevens, B., Kagan, S., Yamada, J., Epstein, I., Beamer, M., Bilodeau, M. and Baruchel, S. (2004) 'Adventure therapy for adolescents with cancer.' *Pediatric Blood Cancer 43,* 278–284.

Stevens-Simon, C. (1998) 'Contraceptive care of adolescents.' *Pediatric Review 19,* 409–417.

Stevens-Simon, C., Beach, R.K. and Klerman, L.V. (2001) 'To be rather than not to be – that is the problem with the questions we ask adolescents about their childbearing intentions.' *Archives of Pediatric and Adolescent Medicine 155,* 1298–1300.

Stevens-Simon, C., Kelly, L.S., Singer, D. and Cox, A. (1996) 'Reasons pregnant adolescents give for not using contraceptives prior to conception.' *Journal of Adolescent Health 19,* 48–53.

Stuart, O. (1996) 'Yes, we mean black disabled people too.' In W.I.U. Ahmad and K. Atkin (eds) *'Race' and Community Care.* Buckingham: Open University Press.

Summerskill, B. (2002) 'Selfish? Miserable? Not us, say UK teens.' *The Observer* 21 July.

Surís, J.C., Michaud, P.-A. and Viner, R. (2004) 'The adolescent with a chronic condition, Part 1: Developmental issues.' *Archives of Disease in Childhood 89,* 938–942.

Surís, J.C., Resnick, M.D., Cassuto, N. and Blum, R.W. (1996) 'Sexual behaviour of adolescents with chronic disease and disability.' *Journal of Adolescent Health 19,* 124–131.

Swain, J., Finkelstein, V., French, S. and Oliver, M. (2004) *Disabling Barriers – Enabling Environments.* London: Sage.

Swillen, A., Fryns, J., Kleczkowska, A., Massa, G., Vanderschueren-Lodeweyckx, M. and Van den Berghe, H. (1993) 'Intelligence, behaviour and psychosocial development in Turner syndrome: A cross-sectional study of 50 pre-adolescent and adolescent girls (4–20 years).' *Genetic Counselling 4*, 1, 7–18.

Sylven, L., Magnusson, C., Hagenfeldt, K. and von Schoultz, B. (1993) 'Life with Turner's syndrome – a psychological report from 22 middle-aged women.' *Acta Endocrinologica 129*, 188–194.

Tan, S.L. (2004) 'Proceedings of world congress on in vitro maturation of oocytes.' Conference abstract. 12.

Tang, G. (1989) 'Bio-psycho-social aspects of gonadal dysgenesis.' *Journal of Psychosomatic Obstetrics & Gynecology 10*, 113–119.

Tasker, M. (1992) *How Can I Tell You?* Bethesda, MD: Association for the Care of Children's Health.

Tates, K. and Meeuwesen, L. (2001) 'Doctor–parent–child communication: A (re)view of the literature.' *Social Science and Medicine 52*, 6, 839–851.

Taylor, E.J. (1993) 'The search for meaning among persons with cancer.' *Quality of Life: A Nursing Challenge 2*, 65–70.

Thaler-Demers, D. (2001) 'Intimacy issues: Sexuality, fertility, and relationships.' *Seminars in Oncology Nursing 17*, 4, 255–263.

Thickett, K.M., Stableforth, D.E., Davis, R.E., Smith, E. and Edenborough, F.P. (2001) 'Awareness of infertility in men with cystic fibrosis.' *Fertility and Sterility 76*, 407–408.

Thomson, A.B., Campbell, A.J., Irvine, D.C., Anderson, R.A., Kelnar, C.J. and Wallace, W.H. (2002) 'Semen quality and spermatozoal DNA integrity in survivors of childhood cancer: A case-control study.' *Lancet 360*, 361–367.

Thorne, C., Newell, M.L., Botet, F.A., Bohlin, A.B., Ferrazin, A., Giaquinto, C., de Jose, Gomez, I., Mok, J.Y., Mur, A. and Peltier, A. (2002) 'European collaborative study: Older children and adolescents surviving with vertically acquired HIV infection.' *Journal of Acquired Immune Deficiency Syndrome 29*, 4, 396–401.

Tomlinson, M.J. and Pacey, A.A. (2003) 'Practical aspects of sperm banking for cancer patients.' *Human Fertility 6*, 100–105.

Toms, J.R. (ed.) (2004) 'Chapter 9.' *Cancer Stats Monograph 2004.* London: Cancer Research UK.

Tonelli, M.R. (1997) 'Ethical considerations in the treatment of cystic fibrosis.' *Current Opinions in Pulmonary Medicine 3*, 420–424.

Tournaye, H. (2000) 'Storing reproduction for oncology patients: Some points for discussion.' *Molecular and Cellular Endocrinology 169*, 133–136.

Tucker, M.J., Wright, G., Morton, P.C. and Massey, J.B. (1998) 'Birth after cryopreservation of immature oocytes with subsequent in vitro maturation.' *Fertility and Sterility 70*, 578–579.

Turner, H. (1938) 'A syndrome of infantilism, congenital webbed neck, and cubitus valgus.' *Endocrinology 23*, 566–578.

Turner Syndrome Support Society, UK (2002) *Turner Syndrome: Lifelong Guidance and Support.* UK: Tyne and Wear.

Ulrich, M. and Weatherall, A. (2000) 'Motherhood and infertility: Viewing motherhood through the lens of infertility.' *Feminism and Psychology 10*, 3, 323–336.

UNICEF (2001) *A League Table of Teenage Births in Rich Nations.* Florence: UNICEF Innocenti Research Centre.

United Nations (1989) *Convention on the Rights of the Child.* Geneva: United Nations.

Ussher, J.M. (2000) *Women's Health: Contemporary International Perspectives.* Leicester: BPS Books.

Valencia, L.S. and Cromer, B.A. (2000) 'Sexuality and other high risk behaviors in adolescents with chronic illness: A review.' *Journal of Pediatric and Adolescent Gynecology 13*, 53–64.

Vanatta, K., Gartstein, M.A., Short, A. and Noll, R.B. (1998) 'A controlled study of peer relationships of children surviving brain tumors: Teacher, peer, and self ratings.' *Journal of Pediatric Psychology 23*, 5, 279–287.

Van Balen, F. and Trimbos-Kemper, T.C.M. (1995) 'Involuntarily childless couples: Their desire to have children and their motives.' *Journal of Psychosomatic Obstetrics and Gynaecology 16*, 137–144.

Ventura, S.J. (1995) 'Births to unmarried mothers: United States 1980–92.' *Vital Health Statistics Series 21. Data on Natality, Marriage and Divorce 53*, 1, 55.

Venturoli, S., Porcu, E., Fabbri, F., Paradisi, R., Ruggeri, S., Bolelli, S., Orsini, L.F., Gabbi, D. and Flamigni, C. (1986) 'Menstrual irregularities in adolescents: Hormonal pattern and ovarian morphology.' *Hormone Research 24*, 269–279.

Vieira, A.D., Mezzalira, A., Barbieri, D.P., Lehmkuhl, R.C., Rubin, M.I. and Vajta, G. (2002) 'Calves born after open straw vitrification of immature bovine oocytes.' *Cryobiology 45*, 91–94.

Vikho, R. and Apter, D. (1984) 'Endocrine characteristics of adolescent menstrual cycles: Impact of early menarche.' *Journal of Steroid Biochemistry 20*, 1, 213–216.

Vygotsky, L. (1962) *Thought and Language.* Cambridge, MA: MIT Press. Cited in Rushforth (1999) 'Practitioner review: Communicating with hospitalised children: Review and application of research pertaining to children's understanding of health and illness.' *Journal of Child Psychology and Psychiatry 40*, 5, 683–691.

Wallace, J.H., Blacklay, A., Eiser, C., Davies, H., Hawkins, M., Levitt, G.A. and Jenney, M.E. (2001) 'Developing strategies for long-term follow-up of survivors of childhood cancer.' *British Medical Journal 323*, 271–274.

Wallace, W.H.B. (2000) 'Late effects of cancer therapy: Fertility.' Paper presented at 7th International Paediatric Haematology and Oncology Conference, 24–26 May, Edinburgh.

Wallace, W.H.B. and Thomson, A.B. (2003) 'Preservation of fertility in children treated for cancer.' *Archives of Disease in Childhood 88*, 493–496.

Wallace, W.H.B. and Walker, D.A. (2001) 'Conference consensus statement: Ethical and research dilemmas for fertility preservation in children treated for cancer.' *Human Fertility 4*, 69–76.

Wallace, W.H.B., Anderson, R.A. and Irvine, S.D. (2005) 'Fertility preservation for young patients with cancer: Who is at risk and what can be offered?' *Lancet Oncology 6*, 209–218.

Wallace, W.H.B., Thomson, A.B. and Kelsey, T.W. (2003) 'The radiosensitivity of the human oocyte.' *Human Reproduction 18*, 1, 117–121.

Warne, G.L., Grover, S., Hutson, J., Sinclair, A., Metcalfe, S., Northam, E., Freeman, J. and others in the Murdoch Children's Research Institute Sex Study Group (MRCRISSG) (2005) *Journal of Pediatric Endocrinology & Metabolism 18*, 555–567.

Weigers, M.E., Chesler, M.A., Zebrack, B.J. and Goldman, S. (1998) 'Self-reported worries among long-term survivors of childhood cancer and their peers.' *Journal of Psychosocial Oncology 16*, 2, 1–24.

Weinman, J. (1997) *An Outline of Psychology as Applied to Medicine.* Oxford: Butterworth Heinemann.

Werbner, P. (1997) 'Introduction: The dialectics of cultural hybridity.' In P. Werbner and T. Modood (eds) *Debating Cultural Hybridity: Multicultural Identities and the Politics of Anti-Racism.* London/New Jersey: Zed Books.

Westcott, H.L. and Jones, D.P.H. (1999) 'Annotation: The abuse of disabled children.' *Journal of Child Psychology and Psychiatry 40*, 4, 497–506.

Whincup, P.H., Gilg, J.A., Odoki, K., Taylor, S.J.C. and Cook, D.G. (2001) 'Age of menarche in contemporary British teenagers: Survey of girls born between 1982 and 1986.' *British Medical Journal 322*, 1095–1096.

Wide Boman, U., Bryman, I., Halling, K. and Mollers, A. (2000) 'Women with Turner syndrome: Psychological well-being, self-rated health, and social life.' In U. Wide Boman *Turner Syndrome: Psychological and Social Aspects of a Sex Chromosome Disorder*. Goteborg: Goteborg University, Institute for the Health of Women and Children.

Wiener, L.S., Battles, H.B. and Heilman, N. (1998) 'Factors associated with parents' decision to disclose their HIV status diagnosis to their children.' *Child Welfare LXXVII*, 2, 115–135.

Wiener, L.S., Battles, H.B. and Heilman, N. (2000) Public disclosure of a child's HIV infection: Impact on children and families.' *AIDS Patient Care and STDs 14*, 9, 485–497.

Wijeyaratne, C.N., Balen, A.H., Barth, J. and Belchetz, P.E. (2002) 'Polycystic ovary syndrome in South Asian women: A case control study.' *Clinical Endocrinology 57*, 343–350.

Wilford, H. and Hunt, J. (2003) 'An overview of sperm cryopreservation services for adolescent cancer patients in the UK.' *European Journal of Oncology Nursing 7*, 1, 24–32.

Williams, J.H. (1987) *Psychology of Women: Behavior in a Biosocial Context*. New York: Norton.

Winter, L. (1988) 'The role of sexual self-concept in the use of contraceptives.' *Family Planning Perspectives 20*, 123–127.

Woollett, A. (1992) 'Psychological aspects of infertility and infertility investigations.' In P. Nicolson and J. Ussher (eds) *The Psychology of Women's Health and Healthcare*. London: Macmillan.

Woollett, A. and Boyle, M. (2000) 'Reproduction, women's lives and subjectivities.' *Feminism and Psychology 10*, 3, 307–311.

Wynn, P., Picton, H.M., Krapez, J.A., Rutherford, A.J., Balen, A.H. and Gosden, R.G. (1998) 'FSH pre-treatment promotes the numbers of human oocytes reaching metaphase II by in vitro maturation.' *Human Reproduction 13*, 3132–3138.

Yoon, T.K., Kim, T.J., Park, S.E., Hong, S.W., Ko, J.J., Chung, H.M. and Cha, K.Y. (2003) 'Live births after vitrification of oocytes in a stimulated in vitro fertilization–embryo transfer program.' *Fertility and Sterility 79*, 1323–1326.

Young, B., Dixon-Woods, M., Windridge, K.C. and Heney, D. (2003) 'Managing communication with young people who have a potentially life threatening chronic illness: Qualitative study of patients and parents.' *British Medical Journal 326*, 305–308.

Young, L.E. and Fairburn, H.R. (2000) 'Improving the safety of embryo technologies: Possible role of genomic imprinting.' *Theriogenology 53*, 627–648.

Zabin, L.S., Astone, N.M. and Emerson, M.R. (1993) 'Do adolescents want babies? The relationship between attitudes and behavior.' *Journal of Research on Adolescence 3*, 1, 67–86.

Zebrack, B.J. and Chesler, M.A. (2000) 'Managed care: The new context for social work in health care – implications for survivors of childhood cancer and their families.' *Social Work in Health Care 31*, 2, 89–104.

Zebrack, B.J. and Chesler, M.A. (2001) 'Health-related worries, self-image, and life outlooks of long-term survivors of childhood cancer.' *Health and Social Work 26*, 4, 245–256.

Zebrack, B.J., Casillas, J., Nohr, L., Adams, H. and Zeltzer, L.K. (2004) 'Fertility issues for young adult survivors of childhood cancer.' *Psycho-Oncology 13*, 689–699.

Zeltzer, L. (1993) 'Cancer in adolescents and young adults.' *Cancer 71*, 10, 3463–3468.

Zeltzer, L.K., Kellerman, J., Ellenberg, L., Dash, J. and Rigler, D. (1980) 'Psychologic effects of illness in adolescence: II. Impact of illness in adolescents – crucial issues and coping styles.' *The Journal of Pediatrics 97*, 1, 132–138.

Contributors

Sarah Andrews is Director of Passion Training and Consultancy, UK, specializing in sexual and reproductive health promotion. She previously worked for fpa, the UK Family Planning Association, managing a community education project working with vulnerable young people. For many years she ran a pregnancy testing service. Much of her work has concerned issues of sex and disability, especially learning disability.

Karl Atkin is Senior Lecturer in Ethnicity and Health in the Department of Health Sciences at the University of York, UK, with responsibility for the programme of work on ethnicity and health. A sociologist, his current research focuses on community engagement and genetic conditions, heart failure and palliative care, and social exclusion of minority ethnic populations. He has published on the experience of family carers, young people and identity, disability and chronic illness, the organization of health and social care, and the provision of support to people from different minority ethnic groups.

Adam Balen is Professor of Reproductive Medicine and Surgery at Leeds General Infirmary, Leeds, UK. He has established a multi-disciplinary service for the management of complex developmental disorders of the female genital tract. He also has a large research programme for the investigation of polycystic ovary syndrome and female infertility.

Rachel Balen is Principal Lecturer in Social Work in the Centre for Applied Childhood Studies at the University of Huddersfield, Yorkshire, UK. She leads a Masters course in Child Welfare and Protection and has interests in research with children and the psychosocial needs of children with cancer and their families.

Francine Cheater is Professor of Public Health Nursing in the School of Healthcare, University of Leeds, UK. She is a nurse by background, obtained a first degree in Psychology from the University of St Andrews and a PhD from the University of Nottingham. Her research interests include developing and evaluating methods of implementing change, the promotion of health literacy and health services research.

Jocelyn Childs is a Senior Social Worker in the Department of Social Work Services at the Mount Sinai Hospital, New York, and has over ten years of experience in working with children who are HIV-positive and their families. She is on the faculty in the Department of Community and Behavioural Medicine at the Mount Sinai Medical Center, New York, USA.

Nancy Cincotta is the Psychosocial Director of Camp Sunshine (www.campsunshine .org), Maine, USA, a retreat centre providing therapy programmes for children with life-threatening illnesses and their families. She is on the faculty in the Department of Community and Behavioural Medicine at the Mount Sinai Medical Center, New York, USA, and is a Bereavement Consultant there. She is completing a PhD at the Columbia University School of Social Work and has over 25 years of hospital experience as a clinician, supervisor and educator. Her research interests include the study of hope, end of life issues for children and their families and the impact of end of life work on professionals.

Sarah Clough is a mother of a child conceived through egg donation. She is married to Martin. Sarah has Turner Syndrome.

Marilyn Crawshaw is Lecturer in Social Work and Research Fellow at the University of York in the UK. Her interests include the impact of reproductive health on relationships and in particular the effects of fertility impairment following teenage cancer. She is a member of the UK multi-agency Project Group on Assisted Reproduction, Inspector for the Human Fertilisation & Embryology Authority and Adviser to UK DonorLink Voluntary Information Exchange and Contact Register for adults genetically related through donor conception.

Melissa Cull is the founder of The Adrenal Hyperplasia Network UK, the support group for people of all ages with Congenital Adrenal Hyperplasia (CAH), and Research Assistant in the Department of Diabetes, Endocrinology & Lipids Metabolism at the City Hospital, Birmingham, UK.

Jane Davies is a parent who found out when her son was 16 that he was almost certainly infertile.

Andrew Eichenfield is the Medical Director at Camp Sunshine in Maine and Director of Clinical Services in the Division of Rheumatology at the Morgan Stanley Children's Hospital of New York–Presbyterian Columbia University, New York, USA.

Bridget Farrant is Fellow in Adolescent Medicine at the Centre for Adolescent Health, Royal Children's Hospital, Melbourne, Australia. She is a paediatrician from New Zealand.

Dorothy Fielding is Head of Psychological Services, Leeds Teaching Hospitals NHS Trust and Visiting Professor in the Department of Psychology at the University of Leeds, UK.

Claire Fraser is a freelance researcher. Her areas of interest include research with children and young people, researching sensitive topics, child protection/survivor research and evaluation research.

Adam Glaser is Consultant Paediatric and Adolescent Oncologist at Leeds Teaching Hospitals NHS Trust UK. He has a particular interest in the impact of childhood and adolescent cancer on fertility and has researched and published in this area.

David Green is a Clinical Psychologist working at the University of Leeds and the Late Effects clinic at St James's University Hospital, Leeds, UK.

Jen King is the pseudonym for a woman living with Complete Androgen Insensitivity Syndrome (CAIS).

Elizabeth Loughlin is a Social Worker, Creative Arts Therapist and Dance Therapist at the Royal Children's Hospital, Melbourne, Australia. She also works as a dance therapist in other clinical settings with depressed mothers and their infants.

Allan Pacey is Senior Lecturer at the University of Sheffield, UK, and Head of Andrology for the Sheffield Teaching Hospitals NHS Foundation Trust, with over ten years' experience as a clinical researcher. His interests include the psychology of men banking sperm as well as the effect of cancer therapies on semen quality. He is also a cancer survivor of testicular cancer as an adult.

Helen Picton is Reader in Reproduction and Early Development at the University of Leeds, UK, and is Scientific Director of the Assisted Conception Units, Leeds Teaching Hospitals NHS Trust. She has researched and written widely in this field.

Amanda Rodney is a Research Fellow at the Centre for Research in Primary Care, University of Leeds, UK. She is currently working on a systematic review, looking at the social consequences of sickle cell and thalassaemia disorders.

Dan Savage was diagnosed with testicular cancer while in his second year at Lancaster University where he was studying Fine Art. Having completed a Masters degree in Glass at the National Glass Centre he now works as a freelance artist printmaker working primarily on glass.

Susan Sawyer is Professor Adolescent Health in the Department of Paediatrics, the University of Melbourne, Australia. She is Director of the Centre for Adolescent Health at the Royal Children's Hospital and Research Fellow at the Murdoch Childrens Research Institute, Australia.

Mary Self is a psychiatrist working in the Department of Liaison Psychiatry at the University Hospital of Wales, Cardiff, UK. She is a long-term survivor of osteosarcoma and a mother of two children. Her research interests are in the psychological sequelae of cancer and post-traumatic growth. She has written and spoken widely about her cancer experiences.

Brad Zebrack is Assistant Professor of Social Work at the University of Southern California, USA, a former paediatric oncology social worker and a long-term survivor of Hodgkin's lymphoma. His research interests include the impact of cancer on families and quality of life in long-term survivors of childhood cancer and he serves on the board of directors for the Association for Oncology Social Workers as chair of the Social Workers in Oncology Research Group.

Subject Index

Numbers in *italics* refer to tables and figures.

Author Index